ARTHRITIS:
Questions You Have ... Answers You Need

Other titles in this series:

By the same author:

ARTHRITIS:

Questions You Have ... Answers You Need

Ellen Moyer

Consultant editor Dr Robert Youngson

Thorsons
An Imprint of HarperCollins Publishers

Thorsons
An Imprint of HarperCollins*Publishers*
77–85 Fulham Palace Road,
Hammersmith, London W6 8JB
1160 Battery Street,
San Francisco, California 94111–1213

Published by Thorsons 1997
3 5 7 9 10 8 6 4 2

© The People's Medical Society 1993, 1997

The People's Medical Society asserts the moral right to
be identified as the author of this work

A catalogue record for this book
is available from the British Library

ISBN 0 7225 3309 8

Printed and bound in Great Britain by
Caledonian Book Manufacturing Ltd, Glasgow

CONTENTS

PUBLISHER'S NOTE

No popular medical book, however detailed, can ever be considered a substitute for consultation with, or the advice of, a qualified doctor. You will find much in this book that may be of the greatest importance to your health and wellbeing, but the book is not intended to replace your doctor or to discourage you from seeking his or her advice.

If anything in the book leads you to suppose that you may be suffering from the conditions with which it is concerned, you are urged to see your doctor without delay. Every effort has been made to ensure that the contents of this book reflect current medical opinion and that it is as up to date as possible, but it does not claim to contain the last word on any medical matter.

Terms printed in **boldface** can be found in the Glossary, beginning on *page 183*. Only the first mention of the word in the text will be boldfaced.

INTRODUCTION

More than 20 million people in Britain suffer at least one episode of arthritic pain each year. Five million of them suffer from various degrees of osteoarthritis and about half a million have rheumatoid arthritis. The totality of pain and disability from these figures defies the imagination.

The majority of these sufferers are elderly people – arthritis worsens steadily with increasing age – and many of them suffer uncomplainingly and patiently, often unaware of the relief that modern medical treatment can afford them.

Regrettably, although there have been notable scientific advances in the understanding of the condition, there is still no cure for the principal forms of arthritis – osteoarthritis and rheumatoid arthritis. But this does not mean that nothing can be done to improve the quality of life for those who are afflicted by these and other arthritic disorders. In fact, as this book will show, a great deal can be done to relieve symptoms and even to delay the progress of these painful conditions.

A good deal, too, can be done for the morale of people with arthritis, not least by showing the immense amount of research that is currently devoted to these diseases and by outlining the progress that is being made and the promise for the future. You will find in this book an account of most of the important lines of research and advances.

Because there is, so far, no cure, arthritis treatment is often associated with dubious claims and even obvious quackery. So-called remedies which have no chance of proving effective are advertised and sold to unsuspecting people. Money, and worse still, fervent hopes are being thrown away every day in the interests of unscrupulous or sometimes self-deluded vendors of alleged remedies. Without guidance, it is often difficult for untrained people to distinguish the rubbish from the reputable. This book also provides that guidance.

Arthritis: Questions You Have ... Answers You Need is essential reading for anyone who has arthritis

Dr R. M. Youngson, Series Editor
London, 1997

CHAPTER ONE

WHAT'S GOING ON INSIDE THIS JOINT?

Q Let's start at the very beginning. What exactly is arthritis?

A *Arthro* is the Greek word for joint, and *itis* means inflammation. So, simply, arthritis is **inflammation** of a joint, or several joints. Some forms of arthritis inflame more than just joints, however, and at least one form of arthritis, **osteoarthritis**, may cause very little inflammation.

Q What exactly is osteoarthritis? And what other kinds of arthritis are common?

A Briefly, because we'll go into this in more detail soon, osteoarthritis can be thought of as 'wear-and-tear' arthritis, usually caused by joint injuries or old age, and is the most common type of arthritis.

Both **rheumatoid arthritis** and **gout** are also fairly common. Rheumatoid arthritis involves joint inflammation and frequently affects the whole body. Gout involves one or a few inflamed joints, and occurs when **uric acid crystals** form in a joint.

Q **Could you explain what inflammation is?**
A Most of the time, inflammation is the body's protective
   response to an injury or infection. The classic signs –
   heat, redness, swelling and pain – are produced as a
   result of biochemicals secreted by the body's infection-
   fighting immune cells as they attempt to wall off and
   destroy germs and to break down and remove
   damaged tissue. Usually, once the battle is won, inflammation subsides.

   Inflammation can also occur, when for reasons not
   clearly understood, the body's immune system turns
   renegade and attacks its own tissues. This seems to be
   what happens with rheumatoid arthritis. Some
   researchers think it takes both a genetic tendency and
   exposure to a virus or other 'bug' to initiate this
   immune-system change.

Q **So there is inflammation with rheumatoid arthritis and
   other rheumatic diseases, right?**
A Both **acute** (sudden and severe) and **chronic** (ongoing)
   inflammation are possible with rheumatoid arthritis and
   other **rheumatic diseases**. Osteoarthritis, on the other
   hand, may cause only mild inflammation or none at all.

Q **I know that joints include the knees, hips, knuckles,
   and the like. Are there other joints as well?**
A Anywhere in the body where two or more bones meet
   is considered a joint. Most but not all joints allow the
   body to move, bend, even twist and turn to some extent.
   Some joints, such as those between the vertebrae in

the back, are designed to be very strong and allow only slight movement. Others – those in the wrists, for instance, and the other joints in the arms and legs – are quite flexible.

There are hundreds of joints in the body. Besides letting us walk and talk, joints help us to breathe. The joints connecting the ribs to the breast bone (**sternum**) and spine allow the chest to expand when a person inhales. There are also joints in the skull (saw-toothed suture joints which harden once the brain reaches its full size), the middle ear (where they allow three tiny bones to vibrate), even where the roots of the teeth are embedded in the jawbone.

Q **Can arthritis be developed in any joint?**
A Arthritis doesn't normally strike every joint, but there are a lot of places where it can settle. And different forms of arthritis tend to attack different joints. Osteoarthritis seems to target the hips, knees and hands, for instance, while gout – another form of arthritis – often zeroes in on the big toes. This is a very general look at the joints affected by arthritis; later we'll elaborate on the specific forms of arthritis and their manifestations.

By the way, doctors often use the term **articular** in reference to a joint. The term simply means 'relating to joints' – nothing more. Don't let a fancy term like *periarticular* throw you, either. This sounds impressive but just means 'around the joint'. And the prefix *arthro-* or *arthr-* at the beginning of a word also simply refers to a joint or joints.

Q **What holds a joint together? Muscles?**

A Muscles and **tendons** (which connect muscles to bone) play a mainly minor role in keeping joints stable. Actually, **ligaments** – strong, **fibrous** bands which connect bone to bone – wrap around joints like a nest of elastic bands and keep them stable.

Take the knee, for instance. It has four ligaments which are rather well known, at least to football players and even amateur athletes who land hard the wrong way. There is a collateral ligament on either side of the knee and two that cross over inside the joint. But six additional, lesser-known ligaments also hold the knee together.

The structure of some bones helps hold joints together, too. For instance, both the hips and shoulders have a ball-and-socket design which allows these joints to rotate.

Q **So what keeps the bones from grinding against each other like a mortar and pestle?**

A In a healthy joint, the ends of both bones are covered with tough, rubbery, supersmooth tissue called **cartilage**. Cartilage allows bones to glide past one another with little friction.

In addition to cartilage, each joint is encased in a tough, fibrous, fluid-filled **joint capsule**. The cells lining the inside of the capsule form the **synovial membrane**, or **synovium**. These cells perform a vital function. They secrete **synovial fluid**, which is to the joints what oil is to a car's engine. Synovial fluid provides protective lubrication to the joint and helps to nourish the cartilage. Synovial cells are seriously and permanently altered by rheumatoid arthritis.

Q How can I get a visual sense of what a joint looks like?
A The next best thing to seeing a live one is to consult a good anatomy book. We suggest *Anatomy of the Human Body* by Henry Gray. Human anatomy hasn't changed since this book was first published and you can rely on its accuracy. And in the mean time, take a look at the drawing of a typical knee joint, below.

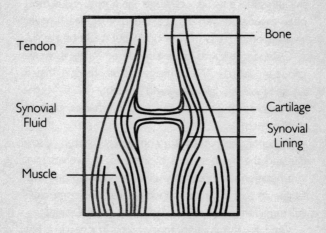

Tendon

Bone

Synovial
Fluid

Cartilage

Synovial
Lining

Muscle

CHAPTER TWO

JOINTS GONE BAD

Q You've briefly described three types of arthritis – osteoarthritis, rheumatoid arthritis and gout. But what are they precisely and how do they differ?

A Osteoarthritis involves the breakdown of that slippery-smooth surface tissue – cartilage – in a joint, and is most often associated with old age and joint injuries. It never involves other parts of your body, but it can be painful.

Osteoarthritis was once considered solely a 'wear-and-tear' disorder. Now most doctors believe that it doesn't have a single cause and probably results from a combination of genetics and joint mechanics, such as misalignment.

Rheumatoid arthritis is a completely different disorder and the more serious of the two. It involves joint inflammation and breakdown, whole-body symptoms of fatigue, loss of appetite and weight loss, and sometimes inflammation in parts of the body besides the joints.

Gout is inflammation and swelling in one or a few joints – usually the toes, but sometimes other joints, too. The inflammation is caused by the formation of tiny needle-shaped crystals in the synovial fluid. These crystals are the result of a build-up of uric acid in the fluid. Gout is the result of various inherent biochemical problems which cause the body to produce excess uric acid. Too much of certain foods and wine that produce uric acid can, of course, make things worse. It is easily treated with a number of drugs, including **colchicine**.

Q **Whom should I turn to if I suspect I have any one of these diseases?**

A Even if you suspect one particular type or the other, it may be best to talk with your family doctor first, before you attempt any self-diagnosis. Your doctor may be able to diagnose and treat you, especially if you have only mild osteoarthritis. Or he or she may send you to a **rheumatologist**, a doctor who specializes in diagnosing and treating arthritis and other rheumatic diseases. We'll talk more about rheumatologists later, but we should mention now that arthritis patients say that these specialists are usually very helpful.

Q **How does a doctor figure out whether I have arthritis?**

A First, he or she has to determine if indeed you have arthritis by ruling out other possible conditions that could cause similar symptoms. Is it possible you could have a joint injury – torn cartilage, for instance – or a muscle or ligament injury? Or maybe you have some other type of inflammation, such as **bursitis** or **tendinitis**? A bone tumour? A fracture?

If it's none of the above, there's more of a chance

that you actually do have arthritis. The doctor's next task is to figure out what kind of arthritis you have. Initially, he or she needs to distinguish between osteoarthritis and some sort of rheumatoid disease, including rheumatoid arthritis.

If it seems that you have rheumatoid arthritis or some other sort of inflammatory arthritis, the next step is to try to pinpoint the type. Is it gout? Rheumatoid arthritis? **Lyme disease** – an increasingly prevalent tick-transmitted form of arthritis? Or maybe even **fibromyalgia**, an ache-all-over condition that is frequently mistaken for Lyme disease these days?

In the early stages of arthritis, it's not always easy to tell just what's happening and what's causing your problem. One thing is important, though. Your doctor needs to make sure you don't have an infected joint – yet another type of arthritis is **infectious arthritis** – because an infected joint needs to be treated promptly with antibiotics. And he or she should be sure you don't have Lyme disease, because that, too, needs to be treated promptly with antibiotics to prevent you from developing unpleasant complications later on.

Q **How does my doctor do all this?**
A Your doctor should first ask a lot of questions about your pain. Remember that your answers can provide valuable clues, so try to be as specific, detailed and accurate as possible. When did it start? What were you doing when you first noticed the discomfort or pain? Has the joint ever been injured? Does it hurt more

when you move it a certain way or when you've been putting pressure on it for a while? Does it seem to snap, grind or lock when you try to move it? Does it hurt even while you're resting? Is it swollen, red, stiff? Do you have other symptoms? Fatigue? Fever? Weight loss? Have you had any recent infections? Any mysterious rashes? Bowel problems? Do you have a family history of arthritis?

Q   **What about a physical examination?**
A   Your doctor will examine your joints, feel around them and move them or have you move them as far as you can. Since several diseases mimic rheumatoid arthritis in its early stages, your doctor may want to do a complete physical examination.

Based on your answers to questions and the findings on examination, your doctor will probably want to carry out some tests. Probably x-rays to look for joint damage, and some blood tests to find out if you do indeed have inflammation present somewhere in your body.

If your doctor thinks you have an infected joint or gout, he or she will withdraw some fluid from that joint to examine for bacteria or for the uric acid crystals that cause gout. Your doctor might also order a blood test for Lyme disease. We'll go into more detail on specific diagnostic tests later.

Q   **There seem to be many forms of arthritis. Is that true?**
A   Certainly. More than 100 conditions belong in the family of what doctors call rheumatic diseases, which involve

inflammation and degeneration of **connective tissue** and related structures. These diseases can affect the joints and other connective tissues in the body, including the muscles, tendons and ligaments, heart and lungs, skin and eyes, as well as the protective coverings of some internal organs.

The family tree of rheumatic diseases includes the types of arthritis we've already mentioned plus some others, especially **systemic lupus erythematosus**, or simply lupus, a chronic inflammation of tissues and organs; and **scleroderma**, a condition that involves thickening of the skin and changes in blood vessels and the immune system. Although many connective tissue diseases are potentially life-threatening, most respond to medical treatment.

Q   **How many people have arthritis?**

A   Many, unfortunately. In Britain, about one third of the population – some 20 million people – suffer some kind of rheumatic complaint each year, and about a million people are significantly affected, long term. As many as 40 per cent, perhaps more, of all people over the age of 65 in Britain have some degree of rheumatic disorder. Five million people have osteoarthritis and half a million have rheumatoid arthritis. It is estimated that 10 per cent of all consultations with GPs are concerned with rheumatic disorders.

Q   **Do only old people get arthritis?**

A   No. Although the incidence of osteoarthritis starts to

increase steadily in people aged 45 or older, rheumatoid arthritis tends to hit people between the ages of 35 and 50. Lupus usually affects women of childbearing age. Lyme disease can strike anyone. **Ankylosing spondylitis**, a condition which leads to stiffening of the spine, occurs most frequently in men aged 16 to 35. And, as its name implies, **juvenile rheumatoid arthritis** affects children.

Q **Who's more likely to get arthritis – women or men?**
A That depends on the type of arthritis. Women are three times more likely than men to develop rheumatoid arthritis and nine times more likely to develop lupus. They're also the primary victims of scleroderma. But men are three times more likely to develop ankylosing spondylitis, and they have a virtual monopoly on gout.

    Osteoarthritis is pretty much an equal-opportunity disease. Men are only slightly less likely to get it than women.

Q **Which joints are most likely to be affected by arthritis?**
A Again, that depends on the type of arthritis. Osteoarthritis can affect any joint, but it commonly occurs in the hips, knees, feet and spine. It can also affect some finger joints, the joint at the base of the thumb, and the joint at the base of the big toe. It rarely affects the wrists, elbows, shoulders, ankles or jaw, unless the joint has been injured.

    Rheumatoid arthritis may first cause pain in your hands, wrists, feet or knees. It can also affect your elbows, shoulders, neck, hips and ankles and, less commonly, just about any other joint, including the jaw.

Gout has a well-known reputation for settling in the big toe, but it can also occur in the hands, wrists, knees, elbows or instep of the foot.

Ankylosing spondylitis, as the name implies, affects the spine, usually starting around the **sacroiliac joints** causing lower-back and hip pain and stiffness. It can also inflame and stiffen the fibrous cords that connect the ribs to the spine and to the breastbone, making it hard to take deep breaths. Also sometimes affected are the heels, making it uncomfortable to stand on hard surfaces.

Q **All this sounds unpleasant, but does it get any worse? Does arthritis cripple people?**

A It can, but for most people it doesn't have to. With proper medical care, including joint replacement and some lifestyle adjustments (walking instead of jogging, for instance, or using a low stool instead of kneeling), most people with arthritis can continue to work, play, reproduce and take care of themselves and their families, although they may have some difficulty and pain doing so.

Studies show that after 10 to 12 years with rheumatoid arthritis, less than 20 per cent of its sufferers are free of disability or deformity. On a cheerier note, of those who do develop such problems, studies show that very few are using wheelchairs or are unable to take care of themselves. Most function independently, even though they have some difficulty performing some daily tasks.

OSTEOARTHRITIS

Q   **Can you give me some more details about osteo-arthritis?**

A   As we said earlier, osteoarthritis is sometimes called wear-and-tear arthritis, or **degenerative joint disease**. It involves the breakdown of cartilage and other tissues in a joint.

Osteoarthritis, or OA, is considered a chronic disease, as are rheumatoid arthritis and most other rheumatic diseases.

Q   **Doesn't chronic mean you have it for a long time?**

A   Right. Chronic means 'persisting over a long period of time'. Doctors use the word to refer to a disease which tends to stick around, even though its symptoms may come and go. Medical treatments can help to alleviate the symptoms of a chronic disease, such as the pain and stiffness of rheumatoid arthritis, and may even slow its course, but they seldom provide a cure. In other words, available treatments usually do not permanently relieve symptoms or tackle the underlying cause of the disease.

Q   **What do you mean when you say that osteoarthritis is a wear-and-tear disease? Are you saying that if you use your joints too hard you end up with osteoarthritis?**

A   Well, no, it isn't that simple. Some people's joints are good for a lot more miles than other people's. Lifelong marathon runners, for instance, are no more likely to develop osteoarthritis than anyone else.

Doctors do know that injured joints are more likely to develop osteoarthritis than joints that have never been injured. They also know that people who are overweight are more likely to develop osteoarthritis in their weight-bearing joints (the knees, mostly), presumably because a heavy load damages these joints. And they know that some people develop osteoarthritis at an age earlier than average, and that this is apparently due to a genetic problem which affects the body's ability to manufacture an important component of cartilage.

In fact, doctors are trying to get away from the wear-and-tear concept and are looking instead at osteoarthritis more as a metabolic problem – one where the body can no longer provide the necessary upkeep and maintenance on a joint.

Q **Who gets osteoarthritis?**
A As we said before, people with injured joints, of course, and people who are overweight may develop osteoarthritis, especially at a younger age. So may people with inherited joint deformities (such as bowlegs or a dislocated hip, which can create uneven wear on cartilage) or people whose bodies have trouble making cartilage.

But just about anyone who lives long enough can expect to have some osteoarthritis. It's one of the oldest and most common diseases known to humanity. It even affects animals.

Q   **What are the symptoms of osteoarthritis?**

A   Osteoarthritis can creep up on you over a period of many years. Many people have mild aching and soreness in their joints, especially when they move. And a few people develop nagging pain, even when they're resting.

The joints tend to hurt most after they've been overused or after long periods of inactivity. It's common to have to work out some stiffness in the morning or after a long period of sitting, by walking and special stretches called **range-of-motion exercises**, which we'll describe later.

In its early stages, osteoarthritis often affects joints on only one side of the body. Rheumatoid arthritis, on the other hand, is usually **symmetrical** – that is, it usually affects the same joint on both sides of the body. And, unlike rheumatoid arthritis, osteoarthritis does not usually cause inflammation of a joint or a general feeling of illness.

Symptoms can be different in different joints, too. In your knees, you may feel a grating or catching sensation. In your hips, you may feel pain around the groin or inner thigh. In your fingers, you're more likely to develop bony growths, called **bone spurs**, which make your joints look swollen even though they're not. Osteoarthritis in your spine may sometimes cause weakness or numbness in your arms or legs.

The pain of osteoarthritis can be severe at times. But sometimes the pain is bad for a year or so, then it lessens, at least temporarily, as the bone ends polish and smooth off.

Q Are all the other joints (apart from the hips, knees, feet and spine) immune from osteoarthritis?

A No. Osteoarthritis can also affect some finger joints, the joint at the base of the thumb, and the joint at the base of the big toe. Rarely, and usually as a result of an injury, osteoarthritis affects the wrists, elbows, shoulders, ankles or jaw. Ballerinas get osteoarthritis in their ankles, prizefighters in their knuckles, and racehorses in their much-abused forelegs.

Q How exactly does osteoarthritis affect a joint to cause such pain?

A There are several stages of osteoarthritis, and in all of them there can be pain. To begin with, the smooth cartilage covering the ends of the bones softens and becomes pitted and frayed. The cartilage loses its elasticity and is easily damaged by overuse or injury. Then, with time, large sections of cartilage may be worn away completely. Without this rubbery, shock-absorbing material, the bones rub together. Which really hurts!

As the cartilage breaks down, the joint may change shape. The bone ends thicken and form bone spurs, where the ligaments and capsule attach to the bone. Fluid-filled **cysts** may form in the bone near the joint. And bits of bone or cartilage that have broken loose may drift around in the joint space, causing pain.

Q How will the doctor determine if I have osteoarthritis?

A He or she will ask you to describe your symptoms and will also ask about any physical stress or injuries that may have led to your pain. Your joints will then be examined, pressed with the fingers, and you will be asked to bend and straighten them as far as you can without pain.

A doctor can usually diagnose osteoarthritis on the basis of a medical history and a physical examination. If there is any doubt about the diagnosis, though, some tests will be required. If you have severe pain in many joints, for instance, or one joint in particular, it's a good idea to make sure you don't have rheumatoid arthritis or some other form of arthritis, or an infection or injury.

Q **So what kinds of tests might my doctor want to do?**
A For starters, he or she may want to x-ray your joints to see if they show the kinds of bone, cartilage and tissue changes typical of osteoarthritis. As we said earlier, joint pain is not always a good measure of joint damage. It's possible to have little pain with moderate joint damage, and some people have a lot of pain with only slight joint damage. An x-ray can help establish the actual amount of joint damage.

If you have a particular joint that's painful, your doctor may want to draw fluid out of the joint to check for infection, inflammation or the tiny crystals that cause gout.

And if you have inflammation or swelling, he or she may want to do some blood tests, including those used to diagnose rheumatoid arthritis. Later we'll discuss these tests in detail.

Q **Is there any way to prevent osteoarthritis?**

A There are several things you can do to lower your risk of developing osteoarthritis:

- Keep to your ideal weight, to protect your knees and hips.
- Avoid sports that commonly result in injury – football, for instance. If you're playing contact sports, wear appropriate protective gear.
- Always wear a seat belt when driving. If your knees hit the dashboard in an accident, later osteoarthritis is highly likely.
- Take regular exercise of a kind appropriate to your body type and level of fitness. Don't jog if you are seriously overweight or have bad knees, for instance.
- Try to adjust your work habits so that you spare your joints. Use a low stool rather than kneeling. Avoid work that is likely to involve accidents or injury.

RHEUMATOID ARTHRITIS

Q **What can you tell me about rheumatoid arthritis?**

A Rheumatoid arthritis (RA for short) is a chronic disease which causes inflamed joints and which can affect other parts of your body, too, including connective tissue and the tissues that surround organs, such as your heart and kidneys. It affects women two to three times more often than men. It can develop at any age, but most often shows up between the ages of 35 and 50.

Q **How can my doctor diagnose rheumatoid arthritis?**

A Diagnosis is easy in people with well-established RA, because they have obvious pain and swelling in symmetrical joints.

Arriving at a definite diagnosis is trickier, however, in people in the early stages of rheumatoid arthritis, when symptoms may be very mild and present in only a few joints. Several inflammation-producing diseases have similar symptoms, and it's hard to differentiate between them and RA.

Just as in the case of osteoarthritis, your doctor will ask you about your symptoms – when they began, which joints are involved, whether you have other symptoms (such as fatigue or fever) and whether you've had any recent infections. Then your joints will be examined and checked for swelling, redness, stiffness and pain. Some blood tests and perhaps some x-rays will probably also be arranged.

Q **Since a certain diagnosis is not always easy to pinpoint, what should my doctor do or look for at the outset?**

A Your doctor should make sure you don't have a kind of arthritis with symptoms similar to those of RA but which needs to be treated quite differently from rheumatoid arthritis.

Infectious arthritis, for instance, which is caused by a bacterial infection in a joint, needs prompt treatment with antibiotics, not **anti-inflammatory drugs**. So does Lyme disease, an arthritic condition caused by the bite of the tiny deer tick. And as we said earlier, a

completely unrelated condition, fibromyalgia, is sometimes mistakenly diagnosed as Lyme disease.

Q **So what tests should my doctor order to rule out
   infectious arthritis and Lyme disease?**
A Infectious arthritis is diagnosed by examining fluid from
   the infected joint, and Lyme disease through a history of
   your symptoms and by a blood test.

Q **Back to rheumatoid arthritis – how does it affect a
   joint?**
A RA strikes the joint capsules of the more flexible joints –
   those in your arms, hands, legs and feet. It inflames
   the normally delicate synovial membrane lining the
   joint capsule, thus affecting its normal functioning.
   This membrane, you'll recall, secretes joint-lubricating
   synovial fluid.

   In rheumatoid arthritis, the synovial membrane thick-
   ens, overgrows and becomes fibrous. It develops folds
   and becomes a harbour for many kinds of immune cells,
   which secrete substances that damage the tissues of
   the joint. Eventually, without treatment, the expanding
   synovium and the misguided immune cells can erode
   away cartilage and **subchondral bone** (bone directly
   beneath the cartilage) and even begin to destroy the
   joint capsule and the ligaments holding a joint together.
   This is called joint deformity, and permanent joint deformity can occur within a year or two after onset of
   rheumatoid arthritis. Although studies have yet to
   confirm it, many doctors treating arthritis believe that

permanent joint deformity can be minimized by early intensive treatment with certain types of **disease-remittive** drugs. We'll discuss this in Chapter 3.

Q   **What causes RA?**

A   No one knows for sure, and there may be more than one specific cause. One popular theory is that rheumatoid arthritis is an **autoimmune disease**, a disorder in which the body turns against itself and begins destroying its own cells and tissue. In fact, there's good evidence to support this theory, including blood tests that show immune-system abnormalities in people with rheumatoid arthritis. Another bit of evidence is the fact that drugs that suppress the immune system improve RA symptoms.

Q   **What makes the immune system go haywire?**

A   This is still uncertain. Many researchers think the disease is due to infection, perhaps from one or more undefined viruses or some other microorganisms, which somehow permanently alter the cells in the joint so that the immune system takes them for foreign tissue and attempts to destroy them. In fact, certain types of arthritis are known to be caused by viral, bacterial or spirochaetal infections, two of which we've already mentioned – infectious arthritis and Lyme disease. But so far, no particular virus or bacteria has been implicated as the cause of rheumatoid arthritis.

Many researchers think it takes a combination of exposure to a virus or other microorganism in conjunction with a genetic tendency towards the disease to cause the immune-system changes typical of an auto-immune disease.

Q **What do you mean by a genetic tendency? You mean if my mother or father had it, I'll get it too?**

A Not necessarily. But if either of your parents or a brother or sister has rheumatoid arthritis, you are three to five times more likely to develop it yourself than someone in the general population.

Q **What if more than one person in my family has RA? Am I certain to get it?**

A No one knows how high your risk climbs if more than one family member has RA.

Q **Can I get tested to see if I carry a genetic tendency to develop rheumatoid arthritis?**

A You would not normally be checked for this genetic tendency unless you were in a research study looking specifically for this sort of thing. Doctors say it's an unusual request, but it may be possible to have your blood drawn and sent to the nearest major laboratory where genetic testing can be done. The test is called HLA (human leukocyte antigen) typing. By the way, the same sort of test is done for tissue matching for organ transplants.

It is true that you can carry **genetic markers** – specific genes – which increase your risk of rheumatoid arthritis and never develop any symptoms of the disease. But there are many other factors involved in developing the disease, and this test is not a particularly useful indicator.

Q   **What exactly is a genetic marker?**

A   It's a location or locations on your **chromosomes**, the genetic material passed on to you from your parents and found in every cell in your body. Certain locations are the DNA sites that determine your hair colour, blood type and many other characteristics. Other sites contain genes that determine a tendency to develop certain kinds of diseases.

HLA typing provides information about a set of genes which influence immune-system function. It can determine if you have genes that may put you at higher-than-normal risk of developing rheumatoid arthritis and other diseases. The test uses certain known proteins, called **antigens**, which stick to receptors on the surfaces of your white blood cells, thereby identifying your particular tissue type.

Q   **Let's say I decide to get this HLA typing test. What is the normal range of genetic markers?**

A   There is no 'normal range' in HLA typing. Instead, the test maps gene sites. Results might look something like 'A2, A12, B4, B8, C2, C4'. The genetic marker HLA-B8 has been associated with lupus, HLA-B27 with ankylosing spondylitis, and HLA-DR4 with rheumatoid arthritis. A rheumatologist or a doctor familiar with genetic testing can explain the results. Among rheumatic diseases, genetic testing has proven most reliable so far in association with ankylosing spondylitis. The genetic marker HLA-B27 is found in nearly everyone with symptoms of that disease.

Q   **What are the more overt indications of RA?**
A   Rheumatoid arthritis is an extremely variable disease – one which can present itself in many ways and which can change and evolve over time. That's one reason it isn't always easy to diagnose in its early stages or to predict its course for any one person.

In about two-thirds of people, rheumatoid arthritis begins with fatigue, lack of appetite, generalized weakness and mild, intermittent muscle and bone stiffness and pain. These symptoms may persist for weeks or months and may baffle both you and your doctor.

Specific symptoms – early-morning stiffness and swollen, painful, hot joints – usually appear gradually, as several joints, especially those of the hands, wrists, knees and feet, become affected, usually on both sides of the body. These symptoms usually come on over the course of weeks or months, but sometimes it can take years for RA to reach its fully-developed form. In about one-third of people, symptoms may be confined to one or just a few joints for months or years. Then more and more joints develop symptoms.

Q   **Don't some people develop rheumatoid arthritis much more quickly than this?**

A   Yes. About 10 per cent of people with RA take only a few days to develop the disease in several joints, often along with fever, swollen lymph nodes and an enlarged spleen. There are no obvious reasons why RA affect certain people in this way. They do not seem to fall into any particular age range, and their genetic markers are much the same as other RA sufferers.

Interestingly, most studies seem to indicate that these people usually do *better* in the long run at avoiding permanent joint deformities than people whose symptoms develop gradually over time. This may, of course, simply be because they get good medical attention and treatment sooner than people with less obvious RA.

Q   **I know you said rheumatoid arthritis can be quite variable in its course, but can you give me some idea of what to expect from this disease?**

A   Expect unpredictability. The disease may take a wide variety of courses. The mildest form of RA is called monocyclic, or one-cycle, rheumatoid arthritis. As its name implies, this is a once-only attack. The person develops rheumatoid arthritis, is treated, gets better and that is that. There are no residual joint deformities or pain. People with monocyclic RA generally have symptoms for no more than a year or two, and sometimes for just a few months.

At the opposite end of the spectrum is malignant RA. People with this kind of arthritis don't respond to treatment, even with the full arsenal of anti-arthritis drugs. They develop joint deformities, usually within a few years of onset of their disease, and end up needing reconstructive joint surgery. Fortunately, only about five per cent of people with RA develop this severe type.

Somewhere in between are the great majority of people with rheumatoid arthritis. Most have symptoms that come and go over many years. Some people's symptoms never seem to get worse. Others have increasingly severe and prolonged **flare-ups**, and start to develop joint deformities. Happily, all these people with the more common manifestations of RA respond to one kind of treatment or another, at least for a time. Their symptoms settle down, or go into **remission** for a time, then flare up, again and again.

Q **What precisely is a flare-up?**
A A period of time when the symptoms of a disease become more severe and obvious. With RA there will be increased pain, stiffness, swelling as well as tiredness and other general features of the disease.

Q **How long can a flare-up last?**
A A flare-up can go on for days, weeks or months. According to experts, there is no particular time frame.

Q **And what is a remission?**
A In a manner of speaking, remission is when your symptoms have gone into hiding. That means that the morning stiffness lasts no longer than 15 minutes, you have no unusual fatigue and no joint pain or swelling,

and blood tests show reduced inflammation. Remissions can last weeks, months or years, but they are seldom total – that is, the sufferer still has some pain.

Remissions can occur in response to treatment, but they can also occur spontaneously, independent of any known cause. No one really understands what causes these spontaneous remissions. Most people with RA have partial remissions. About 5 to 10 per cent of all people with RA go into remission each year, and may stay in remission for a year or so until their arthritis flares up again.

Q   **Does rheumatoid arthritis ever just burn out?**

A   As a matter of fact, there is a condition that's sometimes called 'burned-out' arthritis, although some doctors prefer not to use this term. People with burned-out arthritis no longer have flare-ups, so their joints are no longer swollen. Their blood tests measuring inflammation are close to normal, and they tend not to have the fatigue associated with RA. But they often do have joint pain and disability as a result of their years of having had RA.

Q   **Isn't it true that some people get only a touch of rheumatoid arthritis?**

A   Yes, but they seem to be the lucky few. Some people have only mild flare-ups with long remissions and never suffer much joint damage. When their blood is tested, these people often do not carry genetic markers for rheumatoid arthritis, nor does their blood show signs of inflammation.

Q   **Is there a test my doctor can do to tell if I have rheumatoid arthritis?**

A   There's no one test to confirm that you absolutely and without a doubt have rheumatoid arthritis.

Q   **You've mentioned blood tests several times. It sounds as if a lot of blood testing is done. Is that true?**

A   Well, yes, three blood tests are the standard in the early stages of diagnosis in order to help your doctor get a better idea of what's going on in your body: a **complete blood count**, an **erythrocyte sedimentation rate** test, and a test for **rheumatoid factor** (a protein that signals the presence of inflammation). Furthermore, your doctor can order specific blood tests to check for other types of arthritis or rheumatic diseases, such as Lyme disease or lupus.

Q   **What is a complete blood count?**

A   This test measures a number of components of your blood, including the number of red blood cells (**haematocrit**) and their content (**haemoglobin**); the number and type of white blood cells; and the number of **platelets** (sticky cell fragments that help blood to clot). The complete blood count is the most frequently ordered medical test, and it helps give your doctor an idea of your general health.

Q   **How does it do that?**

A   Let's say you have chronic inflammation, as do many people with RA. In this case the number of red blood cells is usually reduced.

   If you have an infected joint, you may have increased numbers of certain types of white blood cells. These are cells of the immune system which fight infection.

Q   **What is an erythrocyte sedimentation rate test?**

A   The medical term for a red blood cell is an erythrocyte. An ESR, as the test is usually called in the medical world – is a measure of how rapidly red cells sink down to the bottom of a narrow tube. The amount of sedimentation in millimetres is measured exactly 1 hour after the tube is set up. This figure can give the doctor an idea of how much inflammation, if any, is present in your body. This is something the doctor cannot determine merely by examining your joints. This test measures how fast red blood cells cling together, fall and settle to the bottom of the tube. The more inflammatory proteins present in the blood, the faster these cells clump together and sink. So the faster your sedimentation rate, the worse your rheumatoid arthritis may be.

   Keep in mind, however, that a sedimentation rate test simply indicates inflammation. Although it may suggest it, this is not a diagnostic test for rheumatoid arthritis. That's because inflammation can be caused by other conditions besides RA; infections, cancer, even unruptured acute appendicitis can boost sedimentation rates.

Q You also said that another lab test looks for rheumatoid factor. What is rheumatoid factor?

A In simple terms, it's a protein in your blood, one of the
   antibodies, known as immunoglobulin M, or IgM for
   short, which indicates that your body's immune system
   is trying to dispose of other antibodies of the more
   common IgG class.

Q What's an antibody?

A An antibody, or immunoglobulin, is a type of soluble
   blood protein made by the body in response to a
   foreign substance. The purpose of the antibody is to
   bind to the foreign substance and identify it so that it
   can be destroyed by other cells of the immune system.
   But in the case of RA, the body is producing an antibody
   (IgM) to its own antibodies (IgG). The rheumatoid
   factor IgM binds to normal circulating IgG molecules to
   form IgM-IgG complexes, and these complexes are
   deposited in the joints. Once there, they initiate a series
   of immune-system processes which cause the persistent
   inflammation in the joint.

Q So the presence of this rheumatoid factor definitely
   means I have rheumatoid arthritis?

A Not necessarily. Although about two-thirds of people
   with rheumatoid arthritis have rheumatoid factor in
   their blood, a positive test does not necessarily clinch
   the diagnosis. That's because a number of conditions
   besides rheumatoid arthritis are associated with the
   presence of rheumatoid factor. These include lupus,

tuberculosis, cancer and viral infections. And about 5 per cent of all people have rheumatoid factor and no signs of rheumatoid arthritis or any other disease.

Q   So what good is this test?

A   While it's not useful as a screening test, a rheumatoid factor test can be used to confirm a diagnosis in people who have signs and symptoms of rheumatoid arthritis. Also, it can help to identify people who may have particularly aggressive arthritis. The more rheumatoid factor found in a person's blood, the more likely he or she is to have RA that affects more than just the joints.

Q   Is the blood ever checked for other things, too?

A   Blood can be checked for a number of other red flags for inflammation, called *acute phase reactants*. Doing this can give your doctor an idea of the extent of disease activity and the likelihood of progressive joint damage. High levels of these reactants in the blood may make your doctor more likely to recommend early, intensive drug treatment.

Q   My doctor used a needle to draw some fluid out of my swollen joint. Why?

A   Examining the synovial fluid from a swollen joint is helpful in diagnosing a number of conditions, including RA. Your doctor is more likely to do this if only one joint is inflamed. (If only one joint is inflamed, you more likely have a joint infection or gout.) If you've already been diagnosed as having rheumatoid arthritis and have a swollen and inflamed joint which isn't responding to treatment, your doctor may take fluid from that joint to see if it is infected.

Q   **What can joint fluid show?**

A   Joint fluid is examined for its appearance. Normal synovial fluid is a transparent amber colour. If the fluid is cloudy or opaque, you probably have inflammation or an infection in the joint. Joint fluid is also examined for its viscosity, or lubricating qualities. Like oil, the molecules in synovial fluid tend to stick together, providing lubrication. A drop of normal synovial fluid, squeezed from a syringe, has a long, fine tail. Synovial fluid from an inflamed or infected joint does not; therefore, it's a poor lubricant.

Joint fluid is also examined for the number of blood cells it contains. Red blood cells in the fluid may mean the joint has been injured. A high number of white blood cells indicates inflammation or infection. Glucose (sugar) levels are checked, too, and can indicate inflammation or infection.

If it looks as if you have an infection, the laboratory people will take a smear of fluid on a slide, stain it and examine it under the microscope for germs. Microscopy with a special polarizing filter can also show up tiny crystals. If the fluid contains long needle-shaped crystals, you have gout, not rheumatoid arthritis. Some of the fluid will also be put up for **culture** in an incubator. Often helpful because it multiplies the number of micro-organisms, making identification easier, a culture is the growth of bacteria or microorganisms on a special material that provides the microorganism with food.

Q   **Would a doctor ever take a sample of synovial tissue to analyse?**

A   He or she might, especially if you have one joint that is persistently swollen and the doctor is having a hard time figuring out what the problem is, even using the tests we've just mentioned. It's possible to get a bit of synovial tissue using a special hollow-core needle. The doctor carefully inserts the needle into your joint capsule, punching out a plug of tissue about the size of a grain of rice.

Q   **You mentioned x-rays earlier. What do they show?**

A   Early in the disease, x-rays of affected joints are usually not helpful in establishing a diagnosis. They show only what is apparent from physical examination – namely that you have soft-tissue swelling and excess fluid in the joint capsule. However, x-rays can be used to determine if you have bone cancer. This is most likely to be done if you've previously had cancer which might have spread to the bones.

Some doctors take what they call baseline x-rays before they begin treatment. They save these x-rays to compare with those taken later on, perhaps every year or two. This helps them determine the extent of cartilage destruction and bone erosion produced by the disease. Such information can help you and your doctor make decisions regarding drug therapy or even surgery, including when it's time to consider joint replacement.

Q   **What about those fancy, expensive imaging techniques, like MRI? Are they helpful?**

A   In special situations, **magnetic resonance imaging (MRI)** can be helpful, but it's not often used to diagnose rheumatoid arthritis. It's more likely to be helpful if your doctor thinks you have a mechanical problem, such as a dislocation, a misalignment or a ligament or cartilage tear in one of your major joints – the knee, shoulder, hip or wrist. MRI is also very useful in helping a doctor visualize nerve or disc problems in the spine, which sometimes occur with osteoarthritis or ankylosing spondylitis.

Q   **Are other imaging techniques ever helpful?**

A   They can be. **Computerized axial tomographic scans** – CT or CAT scans, for short – can be very helpful in identifying problems in the spine, hips, pelvis and shoulders. The benefit of this technology in this case is that a CT scan provides you with a 3-D image of your bones.

Scans that use radioactive dyes also can provide important information about cell activity within your bones. These scans can detect cells which are rapidly dividing and growing, as they might with cancer, or which are dying off, as they do in some serious bone disorders. The latter condition is called **osteonecrosis**.

Q   So is that about all of the modern technology available
    to diagnose rheumatoid arthritis?

A   No, there's more. **Ultrasound**, a technique that uses
    high-speed sound waves to create images of internal
    organs, is sometimes used to assess joints. The sound
    waves bounce back when they hit solid objects, but go
    through fluids and air. The sound waves are transmitted
    from the tip of a device (a **transducer**) which converts
    high-frequency electrical waves into high-frequency
    sound waves and vice versa. This device is moved back
    and forth over the area to be imaged. The transducer
    picks up the rebounding sound waves, converts them to
    electrical pulses and passes these to an **oscilloscope**, an
    instrument that resembles a television screen, and to a
    receiver which records them on paper.

    Ultrasound can be useful in the detection of soft-
    tissue abnormalities around a joint which are hard to
    detect simply by feeling and bending the joint and which
    may not appear on an x-ray. For instance, **rheumatoid
    nodules** and cysts are best assessed by ultrasound. So
    are tendon injuries.

Q   It seems that a lot of tests are available. How do I
    know if a test is necessary or useful for me? Or must
    I undergo them all?

A   Before you agree to any test or procedure, find out
    exactly why your doctor wants to do it. Informed ques-
    tioning can help ensure that you undergo only those
    tests that are absolutely necessary to pinpoint a diagno-
    sis – an accurate one at that. Ask your doctor:

- What are you looking for with this test?
- What are the possible risks of this test?
- What could be the benefits?
- How long does it take to do?
- Does it hurt?
- What will happen to me if I don't have this test or procedure?

Then, based on the answers and ensuing discussion, make the best decision you can.

Q I have a sense now of how rheumatoid arthritis affects the joints. But you said earlier that RA can affect the whole body. How does it do that?

A First, inflammation anywhere in your body can cause an array of body-wide symptoms – fatigue, slight fever, loss of appetite and weight loss. These are some of the earliest symptoms of rheumatoid arthritis, and practically everyone with RA has these symptoms during a flare-up.

Second, rheumatoid arthritis can cause inflammation not only in your joints but anywhere else in your body. Remember, though, that not everyone with RA develops inflammation in other parts of the body. But some do.

Q How many?

A It's difficult to get a precise number, but it's probably less than 10 per cent.

Q **Will I know if I have inflammation elsewhere in my body?**

A Not always. Many people with this condition never have symptoms. Rheumatoid arthritis can inflame blood vessels, a condition called **vasculitis** which can show up as small brown spots or splinter-shaped marks at the base of your fingernails. Vasculitis can cause a number of serious skin problems. People with RA also tend to bruise easily and to develop small **haemorrhages** under the skin – tiny bluish-purple spots.

Some people with RA develop inflammation around the heart, a condition called **pericarditis**, which can range from mild and fleeting to life-threatening. Chest pain, laboured breathing and swollen feet and hands are the most common symptoms. A very sensitive test to detect pericarditis is an **echocardiogram**, which uses sound waves to detect fluid around the heart sac and other heart abnormalities.

Other complications of RA include:

- lung problems which make breathing difficult
- inflamed nerves (**neuritis**) which can cause loss of sensation in the feet or hands, or muscle paralysis which makes the foot or hand floppy
- **carpal tunnel syndrome**, in which nerves in the wrist are compressed
- eye problems, including dryness, inflammation and pain
- blood and immune-system disorders
- muscle **atrophy**, weakness and tremor

Q **You've mentioned rheumatoid nodules. What are these?**

A Rheumatoid nodules, which develop in about 20 per cent of people with RA, are tender bumps that tend to form at pressure points around joints – where you might rest your elbows on a table, for instance, or around your tailbone. Generally, nodules don't cause pain. Sometimes, though, they become infected and have to be treated with antibiotics or drained.

Q **What's the worst rheumatoid arthritis can get?**

A Well, first the bad news. Rheumatoid arthritis isn't the benign condition many doctors once thought it was. That's partly why they are more likely nowadays to treat it aggressively earlier on. Further, no doctor can predict what's going to happen to each individual person. But they know, from population studies, that after 10 to 12 years more than 80 per cent of people with rheumatoid arthritis show at least some signs of disability or deformity. They can't move their joints through the full range of motion, their walking is slowed, and perhaps they even have trouble maintaining a useful grip.

Q **Is there any good news?**

A Yes. Population studies also show that fewer than five per cent of people with RA become wheelchair-bound or unable to take care of themselves. Most can manage their own affairs, even though they have some degree of difficulty, for example, lifting, kneeling, walking, cooking or holding a pen, paintbrush or comb – activities of daily living. Many doctors believe earlier treatment could help prevent permanent joint deformity, since much of this seems to occur within the first few years of the disease.

Q   **So it's not going to kill me, right?**

A   Very unlikely, but population studies show a tendency for people with rheumatoid arthritis to die a few years sooner than people without RA. The shortened life span, however, is due to a number of mostly preventable health problems.

Q   **What problems?**

A   Infections top the list. Even when not taking drugs that suppress the immune system, people with RA have a somewhat weakened immune system as a result of the disease itself. So they're more likely to develop serious infections, such as pneumonia, which can kill them. They're also more likely than normal to develop non-Hodgkin's **lymphoma**. This is cancer of the lymph glands, which are part of the immune system. This, too, is probably the result of an immune-system disorder.

Q   **How frequently can this occur?**

A   These kinds of cancer are very rare, even in people with RA. They strike fewer than one in 10,000 in the general population, and arthritis researchers think they strike fewer than three in 10,000 RA sufferers.

Q **Any more bad news?**

A Yes. People with RA are more likely to develop stomach and intestinal problems, especially irritation or ulcers caused by anti-inflammatory drugs and other drugs used to treat RA. They may also develop heart or lung problems due to inflammation, and kidney and liver problems, mostly from toxicity to drugs. Probably about 20 per cent of people with RA develop drug-related problems.

Q **But you said there are ways to avoid or prevent the health problems associated with a shorter life span?**

A Annual flu vaccines can help, for a start, as can a regular vaccine against pneumonia.

Other preventive measures are also important, because having to take drugs both for arthritis and for another chronic condition, such as high blood pressure or heart disease, is hard on your kidneys. That means being checked regularly for high blood pressure and high cholesterol levels, and having appropriate tests for early cancer detection, such as mammograms and colon examinations. Non-Hodgkin's lymphomas are usually detected as lymph-node or spleen enlargement during a physical examination, or the development of abnormal proteins in the blood.

Taking preventive measures also means looking after yourself: no smoking or heavy drinking, taking adequate exercise, maintaining a healthy weight, eating nutritiously, and perhaps even taking some vitamin supplements. There's research to show that all these self-care tactics can pay off. If you don't smoke or drink, for instance, you're less likely to develop the ulcers or liver damage that sometimes occur as a side-effect of certain arthritis drugs. If you exercise, your joints stay healthier and more flexible. And if you maintain your proper weight, you're less likely to have painful osteoarthritis on top of RA.

Q **But isn't my doctor supposed to monitor my disease closely?**

A Yes, self-care is just one aspect of the equal-partner relationship you should have with a competent practitioner. And indeed, it is crucial to be monitored by a specialist for potentially serious side-effects caused by any drugs you may be taking for RA.

The next chapter tells you when it's important to see an arthritis specialist, and details the drug and surgical treatments doctors can offer you.

CHAPTER THREE

ARTHRITIS TREATMENTS

Q **What kind of treatments are available for people with arthritis?**

A Drugs, physical therapy, occupational therapy, psychological counselling and surgery are all used to treat arthritis.

Q **What treatment offers the best chance to cure arthritis?**

A There's no treatment that cures arthritis, at least not rheumatoid arthritis or osteoarthritis. Infectious arthritis is another story. It often responds to a single treatment – with antibiotics.

Q **So what does treatment do, if it doesn't cure?**

A Medical care focuses on relieving pain and reducing inflammation, slowing the progress of the disease, preventing permanent joint damage, improving the function of a joint through surgery if necessary, and keeping the patient and his or her joints functional throughout life.

There's no single treatment that accomplishes all of these objectives for any one person. Most people eventually find that a combination of therapies is necessary. For some people, aspirin, exercise and vitamin E work, while for others **gold salts**, hot baths and fish oil do the trick. And for still others, none of these remedies works.

DOCTORS

Q **When should you see a doctor about joint or muscle pain?**

A If your aches and pains are not severe and last just a few days, the chances are that you don't have arthritis. But if your pain persists for more than a few days, recurs over the course of a few weeks or is severe enough to interfere with normal everyday activities, it's time to see a doctor. Swelling around one or more joints usually means there is an underlying problem. So does symmetrical joint pain or joint pain accompanied by fatigue.

Don't be lulled into complacency if over-the-counter drugs such as aspirin or **ibuprofen** keep your joint pain at bay. If you're having to use a painkiller regularly and your pain returns when you stop, it's time to see your doctor.

Q **What happens if I delay going to a doctor for treatment? Will I become crippled?**

A You could. Untreated septic arthritis from an infection in a joint needs urgent treatment if serious damage is to be avoided. An infected joint becomes hot and swollen and requires immediate medical attention.

Q **What about rheumatoid arthritis? Will I become crippled if I delay treatment?**

A Most doctors now think that your chances of developing permanent joint deformities increase the longer you delay treatment. It is now known that permanent joint damage often occurs early on – sometimes within weeks to months of the onset of symptoms. This damage occurs as expanding synovial tissue invades the cartilage in the joint, causing the cartilage to erode. Once this damage has occurred, it cannot be reversed.

This is why many doctors now believe it's important to begin drug treatment early in the course of the disease. We'll discuss this in more detail soon.

Q **What about osteoarthritis? Is early treatment as critical?**

A There's no clear evidence that early treatment helps osteoarthritis, but you can learn some things to help you protect and prolong the life of your afflicted joints. Don't make the mistake of thinking that the way to treat this sort of pain is to 'work it out' – to run up and down stairs or take up jogging. This could be very damaging and could lead to permanent disability.

Q **So seeing a doctor sooner rather than later may be beneficial?**

A Absolutely.

Q **Do I need to see a specialist?**

A First consult your GP. He or she is trained to handle minor illnesses and to recognize a possible serious illness which requires the expertise of a specialist. Watch out, however, for the doctor who fobs you off and does not seem to give your potentially serious medical history the attention it deserves. Research has shown that some GPs may be slow in recognizing the symptoms of rheumatoid arthritis. (We'll talk more about this in a bit.)

Assuming you have a persistent complaint, your doctor should, at the very least, take a reasonable history and examine your joints carefully and gently, check for other symptoms (such as fever and enlarged lymph glands), ask lots of questions about the onset of your pain, and order some of the tests mentioned earlier.

Q **Will my GP be the only doctor I see for treatment? Will he or she refer me to a specialist?**

A Your doctor should refer you to a specialist if he or she thinks you have a serious illness which he or she can't diagnose and treat. You may also be referred to a specialist if your GP is uncertain of the diagnosis.

Q **How can I determine for myself when I need to see a specialist, if my GP doesn't refer me to one?**

A As with many other areas of medicine, you've got to take the trouble to ask questions, stay informed and evaluate your own symptoms and progress.

Ask your doctor:

- What is the diagnosis?
- Exactly what type of arthritis have I got?
- How did you arrive at the diagnosis?
- What makes you think it's this type and not another?

Your doctor's responses to these questions should enable you to decide whether or not the diagnosis was arrived at in a logical manner. If your GP hasn't given you a clear diagnosis within two to three visits over the course of a few weeks, or if you think his or her diagnosis is wrong, it's time to ask whether you can see a specialist. The same applies if your GP has diagnosed your condition but you don't feel better within four to six months of starting treatment.

Q **What kind of specialist should I see?**

A A GP is most likely to refer a patient with arthritis to either a rheumatologist or an **orthopaedic specialist**. A person who appears to have rheumatoid arthritis or some other sort of rheumatic disease is most likely to be referred to a rheumatologist initially. He or she may be referred to an orthopaedic specialist later, if joint problems should develop which would benefit from surgery.

Someone with osteoarthritis may be treated by any one of several kinds of doctors – a GP, a rheumatologist or an orthopaedic specialist. He or she is particularly likely to be referred to an orthopaedic specialist if joint surgery is needed, although an orthopaedic specialist may treat a person with osteoarthritis who doesn't require surgery.

Q **What's a rheumatologist?**

A A rheumatologist is a qualified doctor who specializes in the treatment of diseases of the joints, muscles, bones and tendons. A rheumatologist diagnoses and treats all forms of arthritis, back pain, muscle strains, common athletic injuries and diseases of the connective tissues. He or she may also work closely with other specialists, such as orthopaedic surgeons and physical medicine specialists.

Q **What exactly does the speciality training of a rheumatologist involve?**

A After five years of medical school and a year of pre-registration work in a hospital, the rheumatologist in training has at least three years of specialist training before taking higher professional qualifications and advancing to the grade of senior Registrar. He or she then continues to work in the speciality, under the supervision of a consultant, taking on increasing responsibility. Eventually, a proportion of senior Registrars are appointed as independent consultants.

Q **What is the rheumatologist going to do for me?**

A Because of his or her training and experience, a rheumatologist knows exactly what questions need to be answered and what tests need to be done in order to make an accurate diagnosis. He or she is also very familiar with the arsenal of drugs used to treat arthritis, and so can prescribe them appropriately and monitor their side-effects.

Since a rheumatologist often works with a team of health-care professionals, he or she can help to co-ordinate most aspects of your medical care, including physiotherapy. Rheumatologists are the reigning experts over the whole spectrum of rheumatic disease and over most aspects of its treatment.

Q How do I find a competent rheumatologist?

A The most obvious course is to ask your GP for a referral. And if he or she is referring you to a particular specialist, ask *why* this particular one has been selected.

Q Am I likely to see a consultant?

A It's impossible to say. Senior Registrars and even junior registrars often see patients referred to rheumatic and other specialist clinics. Senior Registrars will commonly take fairly full responsibility for cases, but are required to discuss them with their consultants if any particular problems or difficulties arise. Most senior Registrars are extremely knowledgeable and, because they have recently passed very searching exams, are very up to date. All they lack is long-term experience. Junior Registrars will also usually have taken their higher qualifications in the speciality and will certainly know a great deal more about the subject than any GP or other non-specialist doctor. They are, however, required to work closely with senior Registrars or consultants, who must be kept aware, at all times, of what they are doing.

Q **Rheumatologists can't all be perfect, though, right?**

A No one is perfect. All doctors fall short of perfection from time to time.

Q **How so?**

A Some rheumatologists are said to be less forthcoming with their patients than they might be about the possible side-effects of the drugs they prescribe. They are, of course, fully aware of these side-effects, and many of them take considerable precautions to avoid them. But side-effects such as rashes, diarrhoea, nausea and depression are common and patients are not always warned. Rheumatologists are, however, much too aware of the dangers of more serious side-effects, such as damage to vision from the drug chloroquine, to be casual about them. Patients on high-dose **hydroxychloroquine (Plaquenil)** are routinely referred to ophthalmologists for vision checks.

Many rheumatologists are rather rigidly opposed to the possibility of dietary or nutritional help for arthritis because they think it smacks of quackery. So they're often discouraging to a patient who wants to explore options outside of mainstream medical practice.

And, like all doctors, there may be rheumatologists who are abrasive and impatient. There may even be a very few who are incompetent. But for the most part, rheumatologists score very high when it comes to providing help.

Q   **OK, so now I know something about rheumatologists. What can you tell me about orthopaedic specialists?**

A   An orthopaedic specialist, also called an orthopaedic surgeon, is a qualified doctor who specializes in the surgical treatment of bone and joint diseases, deformities and fractures, including all kinds of problems associated with osteo- and rheumatoid arthritis.

His or her specialist training is along similar lines to that of the rheumatologist, except that a great deal more time is spent in the operating theatre learning the practicalities of orthopaedic surgery. In particular, he or she is trained to repair bone fractures, cartilage tears, injured muscles, tendons or ligaments, and some joint-associated nerve problems.

Q   **It sounds like all this type of doctor does is wield the scalpel. Is that the case?**

A   No, orthopaedic specialists do more than operate, although when it comes to joint surgery, they're the experts. Some orthopaedic specialists do also use non-surgical methods to treat people with arthritis, especially people with osteoarthritis, and can provide a full spectrum of treatment options, including drugs and exercise. It must be stressed that when orthopaedic surgeons are treating arthritis cases they will almost always do so in close collaboration with a rheumatologist. Indeed, nearly all cases of arthritis seen by orthopaedic specialists will have been referred to them by a rheumatologist. Rheumatologists will always prefer a non-surgical solution to a problem if such a solution is available. It is only in cases in which purely medical treatment is inadequate that orthopaedics will be considered and advice taken from an orthopaedic surgeon.

Q **How can I find an orthopaedic specialist?**

A You're not going to have to. If the decision that surgery is required is obvious to you, it will also be obvious to your GP and you will be referred appropriately, either by your GP or by your rheumatologist.

If you and your doctors determine that surgery is necessary, you will automatically be referred to an orthopaedic surgeon known to the hospital rheumatology department, and probably working in the same hospital. Such an orthopaedic surgeon is likely to be operating on many people with arthritis. You are entitled to ask whether the surgeon is one who performs the operation you're to have many times a year, and whether a total joint replacement or shaving off a bit of rough cartilage is necessary. Joint replacement is a highly specialized business calling for very high standards of technique. If your surgeon does only a few joint replacements a year, you may face a higher likelihood of infection or poor fit of an artificial joint. Some doctors recommend that at least 60 per cent of a surgeon's practice should consist of joint-replacement operations. Some experts even suggest 75 per cent as a minimum. There is no reason why you should not ask the surgeon how many he or she does. Be wary of any surgeon who seems to resent this question. Most orthopaedic surgeons perform very large numbers of such operations and will be pleased to fill you in on the extent of their work.

Q **What other doctors treat arthritis?**

A All GPs and many other kinds of doctors may treat one or another arthritis symptoms, so we'll stick with those doctors most commonly used.

A physical medicine specialist is a qualified doctor who specializes in physical medicine and rehabilitation, the medical speciality concerned with diagnosing, evaluating and treating patients with impairments or disabilities that involve the muscles and skeleton, nerves and other body systems. Such doctors are trained to devise preventive or rehabilitative exercise programmes, and are also familiar with non-drug and non-surgical treatments for arthritis. Those treatments include splinting, exercise, water therapy, ice, heat, movement, ultrasound and electrical stimulation. Their principal clinical assistants and auxiliaries are physiotherapists and, to a lesser extent, occupational therapists.

Physical medicine specialists may also use a treatment called *trigger-point therapy*. In this form of treatment a local painkiller or a saline (salt) solution is injected into a painful area of damaged muscle. These injections sometimes stop the pain. They are not used to relieve the pain of arthritis, but are normally limited to the management of the symptoms of muscle and ligament problems, especially in the neck, shoulder and lower back. Many of these problems are, of course, associated with arthritis.

Q **When should I see a physical medicine specialist rather than another practitioner?**

A The answer depends a lot upon whom you talk to. Obviously, physical medicine specialists believe they have much to offer people with arthritis.

Generally speaking, someone whose ability to function has been impaired may benefit from a consultation with a physical medicine specialist. So might people considering surgery on a joint, those with many affected joints, and those having problems using their hands. A physical medicine specialist can devise a specialized exercise programme, use non-drug treatments to relieve pain, and make up immobilizing **splints** for inflamed joints to help prevent permanent damage.

Q **What about osteopaths?**

A Osteopaths are alternative practitioners whose medical training has much in common with that of orthodox doctors. As a general rule, though, they tend to be more holistic than GPs in their approach to care. They pride themselves in the fact that they focus on the patient, not the disease. It is part of their system to view the body as an interrelated system. Osteopaths concentrate on the role of bones, muscles and joints of the body – the musculoskeletal system – in a person's wellbeing. Consequently, manipulation and hands-on diagnosis and treatment are the mainstays of osteopathic practice.

Osteopathic doctors can use palpation (touch), literally a hands-on diagnostic procedure, to detect soft-tissue changes or structural abnormalities. They also use manipulative therapy, in which muscles, bones, joints, nerves and tissue have pressure applied to them in order to effect some beneficial change in a patient's condition. But they will use much the same drugs that orthodox doctors use, if and when such treatment is necessary. Some osteopaths are medically qualified and some have had specialized medical training in rheumatology. People with this kind of background are likely to be highly effective, within the limits of their speciality.

Several surveys have shown that, for many conditions, osteopaths are about as effective as orthodox specialists at relieving arthritis pain. They provide at least moderate relief to slightly more than half of the people they see. People also say that osteopaths are very helpful at providing advice and guidance on exercise and other non-drug, non-surgical alternatives, such as heat, cold and nutritional adjustment.

The principal reservation and concern orthodox doctors have about osteopaths is that they might sometimes undertake treatment without a firm and reliable diagnosis. In conventional medicine, diagnosis is considered an indispensable first step so that treatment can, whenever possible, be directed to eradicating the root cause of the problem rather than just covering up the symptoms. It has to be admitted that, in the case of arthritis, an accurate diagnosis by no means opens the way to definitive removal of the cause and that a great deal of treatment must be directed to treating symptoms. This does not alter the fact, however, that an accurate diagnosis is essential. Regrettably, there have been cases in which osteopaths have continued to treat patients while unaware of the fact that the symptoms were caused by a quite different and much more dangerous condition than was supposed. In such cases, vital time may be wasted which ought to have been devoted to the specific treatment of the real cause of the symptoms – whether it be bone cancer, multiple myelomatosis, or something equally serious.

Most osteopaths are thoroughly alive to this danger and will take great care to be assured of the diagnosis. Some, however, are not so scrupulous. In fairness, it has to be said that the same criticism about treating symptoms without a proper diagnosis can sometimes be levelled at orthodox doctors.

Q **Are there any other specialists I should know about?**
A A neurologist, a doctor who diagnoses and treats disorders of the nerves, may be called in – by a specialist, such as a rheumatologist, or even a GP – to assess nerve damage caused by arthritis. And a neurosurgeon may be called in to perform surgery on your neck or back. He or she might remove osteoarthritic bone spurs on your spine which are pinching nerves in your back, for instance, or fuse together damaged vertebrae to give your spine added stability.

Q   **Well, that's quite a variety of options. GPs, rheuma-tologists, orthopaedic specialists, physical medicine specialists and neurologists, osteopaths – all treating arthritis. Is that the end of the list?**

A   Not quite. Chiropractors and allergists may also get involved, but they are considered alternatives, or adjuncts, to the practitioners we've discussed in this section. We'll explore the options within alternative care in the next chapter.

Q   **Do people spend a lot of time looking for help?**

A   Indeed they do. Nowadays, many people are dissatisfied with the conventional routine of GP and hospital refer-ral and are willing to try to broaden their options. Many who do so find themselves much more satisfied with their level of care. Along the way, however, both patient and therapist are likely to make some mistakes.

Q   **Mistakes? Such as?**

A   We have already covered the main point, namely that many therapists can take a long time to come up with a diagnosis. This is especially true in the case of rheuma-toid arthritis. One study showed that, in one out of five patients with classic, obvious signs of rheumatoid arthri-tis – symmetrical joint pain, morning stiffness and a posi-tive blood test for rheumatoid factor (IgM) – many GPs still took more than six months to reach a correct diag-nosis. In a great many cases the diagnosis was not made until the patient had been referred to a rheumatologist. If this is true of properly qualified doctors, it is likely to be at least as true of alternative practitioners, some of whom have only a smattering of medical knowledge.

Q I'm concerned about this criticism of GPs. Is there anything I can do about that?

A Yes. First ensure that your GP realizes that you think you might have some kind of arthritis. Secondly, let it be clearly known that you are aware that there are different kinds of arthritis. Mention the names. Thirdly, point out that you are aware of the importance of an accurate diagnosis and that you consider such a diagnosis should be made without delay. What you want is not a quick prescription, but proper investigation.

Q Do doctors and other therapists make any other mistakes?

A Once they've finally diagnosed arthritis, the most common mistake some doctors make is to undertreat it – not take it seriously enough to provide effective treatment or suggest a doctor who can. To minimize the harm that might be done as a result of such a mistake, it's important to have medical care from a specialist.

Q Do people with arthritis make mistakes?

A Some patients themselves make the mistake of waiting *years* to see a doctor about their problem.

Q Why would they do that?

A No one knows for sure. It may be that their symptoms are very mild, or that they think their symptoms are an inevitable consequence of growing older, and nothing to see a doctor about. Or it may also be that they seek help outside of orthodox medicine first.

One American study done a few years ago showed that those who stay away from doctors the longest – an average of four years from the onset of their symptoms – were those who were using a non-orthodox treatment. The report did not say if it was helping them, or if they thought there was nothing else they could do, but this was the reason they gave for staying away from qualified doctors.

Q Once again, would you go over the best way for me to get appropriate medical care?

A Here are the principal points to note:

- If you have joint pain or swelling that persists, see a doctor.
- Start with your GP.
- If your GP is unable to diagnose your condition in two or three visits over the course of a few weeks, ask to see a specialist.
- Also ask to be referred to a specialist if the treatment your GP offers has not provided relief within four to six months.
- Ask to see a specialist if, in spite of your GP's treatment, your symptoms get worse.

DRUGS

Q You've indicated that a number of practitioners, notably family doctors, rheumatologists and internists, use drugs to treat arthritis. Is this the primary mode of treatment?

A Yes. In conjunction with exercise and rest, heat, cold and other physical therapies, drugs are a mainstay of treatment for both rheumatoid arthritis and osteoarthritis. Drugs help to relieve pain and inflammation and, in the case of rheumatoid arthritis, may help prevent joint damage.

Q What kinds of drugs are used to treat arthritis?

A There are several different types. Doctors usually divide them into *first-line* and *second-line* drugs.

   The first-line drugs are usually – not always – tried first; they include **nonsteroidal anti-inflammatory drugs (NSAIDs)** such as aspirin, ibuprofen and an array of prescription drugs. These drugs are used for both osteoarthritis and rheumatoid arthritis. First-line drugs used almost exclusively for the treatment of rheumatoid arthritis also include **steroid drugs** such as prednisolone and **cortisone**, although, because of side-effects, these drugs really *aren't* a first choice. Steroid drugs are seldom used for osteoarthritis because they are not helpful for this condition and have potentially serious side-effects.

   Because they are not effective in the treatment of

osteoarthritis, second-line drugs are used to treat only rheumatoid arthritis. They are also sometimes called **disease-modifying** or disease-remittive drugs because their use seems to bring on a remission of symptoms in many people. These drugs include gold salts, as injections or tablets; hydroxychloroquine (Plaquenil), a drug also used to treat malaria; **penicillamine**, a cousin of the famous antibiotic; and **methotrexate** and other **immunosuppressive** drugs also used to treat cancer.

Q **Sounds mind-boggling. How do doctors work out which drugs to use?**

A This is something doctors spend a long time learning, partly by research, partly by study and partly by clinical experience. There are, of course, clear principles laid down in pharmacology textbooks, but prescribing for arthritis is also something of an art. The idea is to decide which drugs will do a patient the most good and the least harm.

Many factors have to be taken into consideration. These include:

- the age of the patient
- the degree of his or her activity
- what other medical problems there are
- whether the patient is willing to take some risks with a newer drug or wants to continue with an older, more well-studied drug
- how he or she has reacted to drugs given earlier
- how the disease seems to be progressing

- what kinds of monitoring tests the patient is willing to put up with.

All these kinds of things need to be considered before the doctor decides how to treat someone.

Some people who have a particularly aggressive form of rheumatoid arthritis at the time they are first seen, for instance, may be put directly on to a second-line drug. Another thing doctors and patients alike need to keep in mind is that a majority of people with arthritis do well on just about any arthritis drug, initially. But after a few years it is not uncommon for the drug to stop working so well, or for it to begin to cause troubling side-effects. In either case, this is an indication for a change to another drug or a combination of drugs.

Q **Well, I suppose it's time I learned something about these drugs. Let's start with the first-line drugs. What are nonsteroidal anti-inflammatory drugs?**

A As the name indicates, NSAIDs are drugs that fight inflammation – pain, swelling, heat and redness. They do that by blocking biochemical substances produced in the body, called **prostaglandins**, some of which cause inflammation. By the way, nonsteroidal anti-inflammatory drugs (NSAIDs) are distinguished from steroid drugs, which also relieve pain and inflammation, by the fact that they work in an entirely different manner and have very different side-effects.

NSAIDs include a few different groups of drugs: aspirin (acetylsalicylic acid) and related compounds such as sodium salicylate, ibuprofen (Brufen, Fenbid, Motrin) and more than a dozen other chemical compounds. If your doctor suggests one NSAID and it doesn't work, he or she is likely then to have you try one in a different chemical group.

Q   **Do you mean that simple aspirin can actually help my arthritis?**

A   As it is not just a painkiller but also an anti-inflammatory drug, it very well might. For many kinds of arthritis, including rheumatoid arthritis and osteoarthritis, NSAIDs are a first-line treatment, and from among these drugs, aspirin is often selected. A great many people with arthritis take aspirin, and they say it relieves their painful, swollen joints. And it's inexpensive, compared with other arthritis drugs.

Q   **How much aspirin would I need to take?**

A   Even though aspirin is available without a prescription, it's important to work with your doctor to determine just how much you need to take to control your symptoms. If you take too much you will suffer the consequences – ringing ears, fluid retention, even internal bleeding. People with osteoarthritis may need only small amounts of aspirin to control their pain, or they may not even need an NSAID at all.

People with rheumatoid arthritis, on the other hand, often need large amounts to control the symptoms of joint inflammation. A doctor may recommend taking three or four standard aspirin tablets four times a day – with meals and a bedtime snack. (A standard tablet contains 325 milligrams [five grains] of aspirin. An 'extra-strength' or 'arthritis-strength' tablet usually contains 500 mg.)

Your doctor should help you to decide the best dosage for you.

Q   **What kind of aspirin is best to take?**

A   Aspirin comes in several forms – buffered and enteric-coated – developed to make them more convenient to take and less likely to lead to some of the major side-effects associated with them, such as stomach distress and ulcers. These side-effects are more likely to appear with the large dosages recommended for people with rheumatoid arthritis.

Buffered aspirin contains antacid-like ingredients which are supposed to minimize aspirin's stomach-irritating effects. Aspirin with a special coating (called enteric-coated) dissolves only when it reaches your small intestine, so the coating saves your stomach from direct contact with the aspirin. Soluble (or dispersible) aspirin is aspirin mixed with citric acid and calcium carbonate (chalk). In water the citric acid reacts with the chalk to form calcium citrate, and this dissolves the aspirin. None of these forms of aspirin offers complete protection from potentially dangerous side-effects, which we'll discuss in a minute.

All forms of aspirin are available in non-brand-name (generic) versions, which work just as well as the popular brands and cost a lot less. Buying a bottle of 1,000 generic enteric-coated aspirin tablets may be the least expensive, least stomach-irritating way to go. A quick tip: to keep the tablets fresh, store the bottle in a dry, cool place – not your bathroom!

The one form of aspirin you should avoid is the original, old-fashioned formulation – a hard, insoluble tablet that is difficult to break. Pure compressed aspirin can be very irritating and damaging to the lining of the stomach. If you remember that salicylic acid is commonly used to dissolve warts on the skin, you will see how strong aspirin can be.

Q   **You said that people with osteoarthritis may not need to take an NSAID. What kind of drug would they take?**

A   Since mild osteoarthritis may involve pain but not inflammation, an anti-inflammatory drug, with all its possible side-effects, may not be necessary. People with osteoarthritis may do just fine taking an aspirin substitute, **acetaminophen** (paracetamol), which is sold as Alvedon, Calpol, Medinol, Paldesic, Salzone and under various other brand names.

In fact, research has shown that people with chronic knee pain caused by osteoarthritis responded just as well to four weeks of treatment with acetaminophen as they did to four weeks of the NSAID ibuprofen. You should be able to judge within four to six weeks whether or not paracetamol is the drug for you. Remember, however, that although paracetamol has few side-effects in normal dosage, overdosage can cause serious and often fatal liver damage.

Q   **Aside from aspirin, what other kinds of NSAIDs are available?**

A   Many different over-the-counter drugs contain aspirin or related compounds. Some contain ibuprofen (Brufen, Junifen, Motrin or Fenbid).

   Many NSAIDs are available by prescription only. Some of those commonly used for arthritis include ibuprofen (Motrin) in dosages up to four times the over-the-counter version, indomethacin (Indocid, Indomod), naproxen (Naprosyn), piroxicam (Feldene), tolmetin (Tolectin) and sulindac (Clinoril).

Q   **Why are these drugs available only by prescription, while some other NSAIDs are not?**

A   The latter drugs have potentially serious side-effects which require a doctor's monitoring.

Q   **Why so many drugs designed to do basically the same thing – relieve pain and inflammation?**

A   One reason is that drug manufacturers are always trying to come up with new drugs that work as well as, or better than, aspirin but have fewer of the side-effects mentioned – stomach distress and ulcers. Another reason is that a large selection provides a benefit: some people fail to respond adequately to a particular NSAID, but when they try a different one, it may work very well.

Q   **But are NSAIDs so very different from one another?**

A   To hear the pharmaceutical companies' talk, you would think so. Every time a new NSAID hits the market, the drug manufacturer seems to promote it as being at least as effective as those already on the market but with fewer side-effects. The truth so far is that NSAIDs on the market all perform in much the same way.

Many claim that there is nothing to beat ibuprofen, but others disagree. Presumably experience varies because of the chance differences in patient reaction. But even well-organized trials tend to give mixed results.

Q **How soon can I tell if an NSAID is working for me?**
A Your pain and inflammation may not be relieved immediately – it may take a while. Generally, you'll spend a week or two gradually increasing your dosage to get up to a 'therapeutic level' – a dosage that maintains the drug at a blood level that should reduce pain and relieve inflammation. Your doctor will probably want you to continue with this dosage for about a month before deciding whether the drug is working for you. If it's not satisfactory, most likely another NSAID will be tried, at least for a time. But if NSAIDs do not seem to be working, most doctors will move on to second-line drugs.

In rheumatoid arthritis, almost all doctors still start off with a good trial of NSAIDs. But these days they are quicker to move on to more powerful drugs. It is not generally considered good medicine to wait until a patient has signs of joint erosions on x-ray before switching to stronger drugs.

Q **I want to know more about the side-effects NSAIDs have. What are they?**

A All arthritis drugs have side-effects, and the NSAIDs are no exception. Some of these we've already mentioned: stomach irritation may occur with just about any NSAID, including aspirin. Other effects include heartburn, indigestion, pain, nausea and vomiting. And about one in five people who take these drugs in large doses or over a long period of time develops stomach or intestinal ulcers, studies show. That's about 10 times the normal rate.

Q **Ulcers – aren't they sometimes serious?**

A Unfortunately, yes. It seems clear that many hundreds of people die from NSAID-induced peptic ulcers each year.

Q **You mean that the aspirin or whatever NSAID I take can lead to a hole in my stomach?**

A They can do, but this is very rare. The real reason the ulcers occur is because NSAIDs suppress the production of a range of natural body substances, prostaglandins. As you'll recall, we said earlier that some prostaglandins can cause inflammation. But other prostaglandins are good; they help maintain the cells that form your stomach lining. Unfortunately, the NSAIDs suppress *both* types of prostaglandins.

Q   **What can I do to avoid getting ulcers?**

A   Three things: be closely monitored by your doctor for early signs of ulcers; reduce related risk factors; and take a drug that helps to protect against the development of ulcers.

Q   **What kind of monitoring should my doctor do?**

A   Every couple of months, your doctor should do a blood test called a complete blood count. This test can detect a decrease in red blood cells, which may mean you are bleeding internally. Your doctor may also have you test your stools for blood. This is a simple at-home test you can do yourself every couple of weeks.

Your doctor should also ask you about stomach pains or any other kind of stomach discomfort – if he or she doesn't, make sure you volunteer the information. Be aware, though, that pain is not always present with NSAID-induced ulcers, since the drugs themselves can mask the ulcer pain.

You can do something in the way of self-care. Contact your doctor *immediately* if you vomit blood or develop black, tarry stools. These are signs of internal bleeding. And check with your doctor if you have severe heartburn, stomach pain that goes away after you eat food or take antacids, severe stomach cramps, or occasional nausea or vomiting for no apparent reason.

Q   **How else can I reduce my risk of developing ulcers?**

A   Don't smoke cigarettes, don't drink alcohol and don't take steroid drugs along with NSAIDs. All three increase the odds in favour of your developing an ulcer.

Q Isn't there a drug to prevent these ulcers?

A   Yes, it's called misoprostol (Cytotec). This unique drug is a prostaglandin analogue – that is, it acts rather like a prostaglandin in stimulating the growth of mucus-producing cells that protect the stomach lining. It is expressly intended for the treatment and prevention of stomach ulcers in people taking NSAIDs. In clinical trials, people taking NSAIDS who also took either 400 or 800 mcg (micrograms) of Cytotec daily had a significant reduction in stomach-lining injury compared with a group taking a **placebo** (a harmless, 'empty' pill). The rate of microscopic stomach injury was 70 to 75 per cent in the placebo group but only 10 to 30 per cent in those taking Cytotec.

   The most common side-effects of Cytotec, diarrhoea and abdominal pain, occurred in about 13 per cent of people. This side-effect can be minimized by taking the drug immediately after meals or at bedtime.

Q What about other, less expensive ulcer drugs? Can't I take them?

A   Some doctors prescribe other ulcer drugs, such as Tagamet or Zantac (histamine blockers which reduce acid production) or strong antacids. These drugs can help to heal an ulcer that has already formed if the NSAIDs are stopped during the two- to three-month healing process, but there is no real proof that they help to stop stomach ulcers from forming.

Q **Apart from causing ulcers, what other side-effects do NSAIDs cause?**

A A few people develop asthma, hay fever, nasal congestion or hives from aspirin or other NSAIDs. If they develop such symptoms, they should avoid taking drugs containing aspirin or related compounds.

Aspirin and some other NSAIDs can slow blood-clotting time, making bleeding a problem. For this reason, these drugs are usually stopped for one to two weeks prior to any kind of surgery.

High doses of aspirin can make your ears ring (tinnitus) and cause slight deafness. This almost certainly indicates that you've taken too much aspirin for your system; you should reduce your dosage and call your doctor. Ringing in the ears is a sign of potentially permanent inner ear damage, and may progress to permanent tinnitus and irremediable deafness.

Aspirin and other NSAIDs – and many other drugs – can cause fluid retention and problems for your kidneys and liver. If you begin to retain fluid and swell up, gain a lot of weight or feel ill while you're taking one of these drugs, stop taking it and call your doctor at once. It may mean a drug is building up to a toxic level in your body.

Q **Is toxicity a common problem with these drugs?**

A It can be a problem for some, especially older people and those taking additional drugs, such as diuretics (drugs that flush fluid out of your body). And certain drugs can build up to toxic levels in your body much faster than others, causing kidney or liver damage.

The percentage of people who develop kidney or liver toxicity varies from drug to drug. There are now a number of good books on the popular medicine market that deal with prescription drugs. You can check these for drug side-effects and toxicity. Alternatively, you could consult the reference department of your local library.

Q **Why is toxicity a problem?**

A One reason, oddly enough, is the enormous variability in the size of patients. Drug dosage ought, ideally, to be related to the weight of the patient. Age also has a bearing on a drug's effect. The only fully reliable way to achieve consistent effects safely would be to monitor a patient's blood levels of the drug. Very few doctors do this. As a result, very small patients, especially women, sometimes get what amounts to an overdose.

Q **What can I do about this problem?**

A Get regular urine and blood tests to detect any kidney or liver damage. If the tests indicate you are developing problems, your doctor should probably refer you to a specialist. At the very least, he or she should change you to a different drug in the same class, at a lower equivalent dosage.

Q **Are NSAIDs the only first-line drugs?**

A No. Steroid drugs are sometimes called first-line drugs, too, but this is something of a misnomer. These drugs are not likely to be the first choice for most kinds of arthritis, and they are almost never used for osteoarthritis.

Q   **Why? Are steroids really dangerous to take?**

A   They can be. Steroids were once given in large doses, for long periods of time, for inflammation-producing diseases such as rheumatoid arthritis. The results were often dramatic, but because they were used in large doses for long amounts of time, they produced many side-effects. These included:

- lowered resistance to infection
- weight gain
- 'moon face'
- bone loss
- muscle wasting
- mood changes
- blurred vision
- cataracts
- diabetes
- raised blood pressure.

These days, for most cases of rheumatoid arthritis, steroids are generally not used in large amounts, or for very long, so serious side-effects are less likely to occur. Still, these drugs do need to be used carefully, to make sure they are not causing any of the above-mentioned side-effects.

Q **What exactly are steroids?**

A Steroids are synthetic copies or variants of inflammation-taming hormones, called corticosteroids and glucocorticoids, produced by the body's adrenal glands. The drugs go by such names as dexamethasone, hydrocortisone and prednisolone.

Q **How are steroids prescribed?**

A Doctors seem to vary widely in how they prescribe steroids. Some are very unhappy about their use in arthritis and try to avoid them when possible; others, although aware of the disadvantages, use them quite a lot. Because oral steroids, such as prednisolone, provide almost immediate relief of pain and inflammation, they may be given in addition to NSAIDs to relieve severe symptoms, especially when both patient and doctor are waiting for a slower-acting drug, such as gold, to take effect. Some doctors also offer their patients steroids to help them get through a flare-up, especially if the patient is the sole breadwinner of a family, so that the person can continue to work. Some, on the other hand, keep patients on low doses of steroids (less than 10 mg a day) for months or years. Patients on long-term steroids may include people who aren't responding to NSAIDs and, especially, people who are at particular risk of developing side-effects from NSAIDs.

Q **How can I avoid trouble with steroids?**

A Most doctors agree that you should take them in the

smallest dose that relieves your symptoms for as short a time as possible.

Further, these drugs need to be tapered off – slowly reduced in dosage – before they are finally stopped altogether. That's because they suppress your body's production of steroids. By reducing the dose slowly, your body has time to come back to normal steroid production.

Most doctors have their patients begin to slowly taper off the drug after eight to twelve weeks of use, or sooner if possible.

Here again, it's important to ask your doctor lots of questions. Why are you prescribing this drug? What are its benefits? What are the risks? How can I minimize the risks? How do you intend to monitor for risks?

Q   How does a doctor monitor for steroid risks?

A   Regular blood-pressure checks, a full blood count and blood tests that check blood sugar. Some doctors also occasionally do an x-ray test to check bone density.

Q   Are steroids only taken orally?

A   No. Steroids can be injected directly into just about any inflamed joint, and usually provide quick relief which may last for months, even years.

Q   Is there an advantage to injections rather than oral steroids?

A   Yes. Injections do not cause the body-wide side-effects, such as bone loss or lowered resistance to infection, that are seen with oral steroids. But many doctors caution that a joint should not be injected more than three times a year. Others recommend no more than once every three months. That's because frequently repeated injections are thought to be capable of leading to joint destruction.

Another word of caution from experts: steroids should never be injected into a joint that's infected, because they can make the infection worse. Your doctor should rule out infection by checking the fluid in the joint for signs of infection before giving you a steroid injection.

Q **Are steroids ever used to treat osteoarthritis?**

A Most experts agree that systemic, or oral steroids, have no place in the treatment of osteoarthritis. That's because osteoarthritis seldom involves severe inflammation, the condition steroid drugs treat best. Nevertheless, some doctors believe steroid injections into a painful joint may be given three times a year in severe cases of osteoarthritis, in cases in which it is obvious that joints will eventually have to be replaced.

Q **When do the second-line, or disease-remittive, drugs come in?**

A As the name implies, a second-line drug – gold, methotrexate and the like – may be added to your treatment if NSAIDs are not working well enough to relieve your symptoms. These drugs are reserved almost exclusively for rheumatoid arthritis and other rheumatic diseases; they are seldom used for osteoarthritis.

Q How do second-line drugs differ from first-line drugs?
A All second-line drugs are slow acting. They can take weeks or months to take effect.

Unlike NSAIDs and steroids, these drugs are thought to slow the progress of your disease. They do sometimes bring on remission or partial remission. In truth, though, there's little scientific evidence to prove that these drugs actually do slow the progress of rheumatoid arthritis. The little proof there is seems to indicate that these drugs have a major impact in slowing the course of rheumatoid arthritis only when they are used early in the development of the disease.

The only clinical trial that supports the theory that second-line drugs can help prevent permanent joint damage was done by Dutch researchers. This study, published in 1989 in the *Lancet*, found that a drug used most often for the treatment of ulcerative colitis, **sulphasalazine**, helped to prevent joint-cartilage breakdown in people with early rheumatoid arthritis.

As for anecdotal evidence, doctors point out that people who have aggressive RA often do better than those with slow-acting RA because they are treated sooner with second-line drugs.

Because of these findings, many doctors who treat rheumatoid arthritis now turn to these drugs earlier than they used to. How soon they decide to do so depends on a number of factors, but especially the stage the disease is at when the patient is first seen. In some cases, second-line drugs may be started immediately. If the risk of NSAID-related side-effects, such as ulcers, is considered to be high, this may be taken to be an indication for starting second-line drugs early.

Q **But why even bother to be treated with these drugs if there is so little proof that they do anything to slow the course of the disease?**

A There is a difference between slowing the course of a disease and improving the quality of a patient's life. No one doubts that the quality of life of many patients is, in fact, markedly improved by these drugs. This area of medicine is one in which the relief of symptoms is wholly justified, even if the underlying cause of them may not be markedly affected.

Q **What again are the most commonly prescribed second-line drugs?**

A These drugs include gold salts, as injections or pills; hydroxychloroquine (Plaquenil), a drug also used to treat malaria; penicillamine, a cousin of the famous antibiotic; and methotrexate and other immunosuppressive drugs also used to treat cancer.

Q **You said gold – do you mean the same metal that's used in jewellery? How does it work in the treatment of arthritis?**

A The pure metal is inert and is not used. But all metals

can be treated with acids to form compounds known as salts; these are soluble and can be used as drugs. Gold salts are the soluble form of the same precious metal used in jewellery, and can be given as injections or pills. The most effective gold compounds for rheumatoid arthritis are those in which the molecule contains sulphur. Gold has been used since the 1920s to treat rheumatoid arthritis, and it works well enough to provide a standard against which potential new drugs are compared to see if they do as well.

Q   **How is gold given?**

A   Gold injections are usually given once a week during the first few months, in slowly increasing doses, then once a month as a maintenance dose.

Oral gold is convenient – no injections! It's usually given as two capsules daily.

Q   **What kinds of side-effects does gold have?**

A   Kidney damage is a possible serious side-effect. To detect early signs of kidney injury, urine tests are done repeatedly during therapy.

Damage to the bone marrow (where the body manufactures red and white blood cells and platelets) is another possible serious side-effect. To identify this complication, blood tests are done from time to time.

An itchy skin rash can occur, too. Generally, the rash is mild and affects only a few spots on the body. Sometimes, though, it can be severe. The rash usually disappears within a few weeks if gold is stopped.

In about 3 out of 10 people, injectable gold has to be stopped because of some side-effects. People taking oral gold are less likely to have the serious side-effects that necessitate stopping the drug, but they still need to be monitored for side-effects. And they're more likely to develop diarrhoea with oral gold than with gold injections. Although oral gold is probably a little safer than gold injections, it's also probably a little less effective.

If either form of gold is going to work, you'll feel a clear difference within three to six months, doctors say. One or two people out of every 10, however, get no benefit from injected gold.

Q Is gold an expensive treatment?

A Treatment with auranofin (Ridaura) tablets currently costs the NHS £28 a month. This need not concern you, however. If you need the drug, you will get it and will have to pay only the prescription charge. This is one instance of really getting your money's worth out of the NHS.

Q And what is penicillamine? How does it work? How is it different from gold?

A This drug, sold under the trade names of Distamine and Pendramine, is known to remove copper from the body. This makes it an ideal treatment for people with a rare illness called Wilson's disease, which causes a potentially fatal build-up of copper in the body. But no one knows what penicillamine does to make it effective against the pain and inflammation of rheumatoid arthritis, or if its ability to remove copper is important in this regard. The drug seems to influence the immune system. Interestingly, it leads to a marked reduction in the rheumatoid factor IgM used to help in the diagnosis of the disease.

In studies, penicillamine seems to work about as well as gold, in the people who can tolerate it. The drug's notorious side-effects, which include kidney problems, rashes, muscle weakness, bone-marrow suppression and severe allergic reactions in people allergic to penicillin, have made it fall out of favour with rheumatologists. Formerly, rheumatologists used it a lot in people who had failed to respond to gold injections or who couldn't tolerate gold. Because of the extent and severity of side-effects, however, its place in the list of anti-rheumatic drugs has been largely replaced by immuno-suppressive drugs, such as methotrexate.

Q And what about the malaria drug you said is also used to treat arthritis?

A This drug is a form of chloroquine, hydroxychloroquine sulphate, sold under the trade name Plaquenil, like gold, no one really understands how it works. Also like gold, it takes three to six months to relieve pain and inflammation. It is probably not as effective as gold, but some doctors like to try this drug before they try gold, because, if it works, patients are likely to be able to stay on it for a long time with few serious side-effects. Plaquenil is one of the safest second-line arthritis drugs.

Q **What kind of side-effects does Plaquenil have?**

A The chief anxiety is its effect on the eyes, but doctors are now using lower doses, which are much less likely to have this effect.

Q **What happens to the eyes?**

A Plaquenil can damage the retina – the cells lining the back of the eye – and it can also cause opacities in the corneas – the front lenses of the eyes. So if you're taking this drug, you need to have your eyes checked every four to six months to ensure that there is no subtle reduction in the acuity of your vision. In general, the total dose of chloroquine taken must exceed about 100 g (that would mean more than 500 tablets of 200-mg strength each) before eye problems are to be expected. It is rare for retinal damage (retinopathy) to occur in less than a year's treatment.

Unfortunately, chloroquine is retained in the body for years after it is stopped, and retinopathy has been known to occur several years after treatment.

Q **What would I actually notice if chloroquine was causing eye damage?**

A Corneal damage causes vague blurring of vision and 'glare' in bright light. There may be a coloured halo around lights. Happily, the effect on the cornea is completely reversible and will clear spontaneously when the drug is stopped. The same cannot be said for the effect on the retina. This is a severe degenerative change that can progress to complete blindness.

Examination of the retinas with an ophthalmoscope can reveal the characteristic pigmentary changes. As far as the affected person is concerned, there is a gradual deterioration in the clarity and sharpness of vision which cannot be improved by any change of glasses.

Q **Now, about these immunosuppressive drugs you've been talking about – what do they do?**

A These drugs make your immune system a little less lively, so, in the case of rheumatoid arthritis, the renegade immune cells which are nibbling at your joints, back off a bit. Unfortunately, these drugs affect your *entire* immune system, increasing your risk of developing serious infections. Plus, they have other potentially life-threatening side-effects.

The most popular of these drugs, methotrexate, was first used experimentally to treat rheumatoid arthritis in 1951. But it wasn't until recently, after many years of study, that rheumatologists started using methotrexate with some frequency. Immunosuppressive drugs were first used, in doses hundreds of times larger, to treat cancer. They are also used to prevent the rejection of transplanted organs and to treat otherwise uncontrollable cases of the persistent skin disease psoriasis.

Q **When is methotrexate used for rheumatoid arthritis instead of gold or Plaquenil, the antimalaria drug?**

A Some doctors try methotrexate on patients who have not improved on gold or Plaquenil. Others may suggest either methotrexate or gold injections to a patient and, after explaining fully the risks and benefits, let the patient decide which to have. At one time there was a fairly rigid order of priority for their use, but doctors now take a more flexible view of the matter. Any doctor prescribing an immunosuppressive drug early in the management of a case of rheumatoid arthritis would, of course, carefully explain the risks. This, together with the other second-line drugs, is not a form of treatment that can be given without the patient's informed consent.

Q **What are the risks and benefits of methotrexate, compared with gold injections?**

A Both these drugs have potentially serious – even fatal – side-effects, and require careful monitoring. Gold injections, for instance, or penicillamine containing even a trace of penicillin, may on rare occasions cause a potentially fatal allergic reaction called anaphylactic shock. Methotrexate can cause unexpectedly severe and sometimes fatal bone-marrow suppression and gastrointestinal toxicity, usually in people who are taking steroid drugs at the same time.

Gold is more likely than methotrexate to cause kidney damage; but methotrexate is more likely than gold to cause liver damage. Gold, not methotrexate, is likely to be prescribed to heavy drinkers. Both drugs can cause serious changes in the blood which may require stopping their use, and both can cause birth defects if given to pregnant women. Both, too, have an array of bothersome side-effects, such as skin rashes, nausea, loss of appetite and headaches.

Gold begins to work more slowly than methotrexate. People taking gold may begin to see improvement only after three to six months of treatment; people taking methotrexate may see improvement in one to two months.

About 80 per cent of the people taking injected gold see an improvement in symptoms, but about one-third of them have to stop taking gold at some point because of the side-effects. About 80 per cent of the people taking methotrexate respond initially. And about 50 per cent of people are still taking the drug with no problems five years after they start. Stopping either drug can lead to a flare-up.

Because gold has been used so much longer than methotrexate, there are no surprises about its risks and benefits, including its possible long-term effects. With methotrexate, this is not the case. Many doctors say we won't know this drug's real benefits – or risks – for another 10 years or more.

Q In what percentage of cases is methotrexate effective?
A Studies show that about half of the people who take methotrexate get significant relief from their joint pain and swelling.

Q How is methotrexate given?
A Usually, it's given in tablet form about once every 10 days. Sometimes it's given by weekly injections. And, as we already mentioned, methotrexate seems to start working faster than gold: benefits are seen in one to two months.

Q How long do I have to take this drug?

A   Like other arthritis drugs, this is a long-term treatment. People may improve steadily over successive months, but if they stop taking the drug they're likely to have a major flare-up within a few weeks. Some people have now been taking methotrexate for 10 years or longer with no serious side-effects.

Q What kind of side-effects do you need to watch out for with this drug?

A   The most common side-effect is nausea, which can be minimized by spreading your dose out over the day you take it. More troubling side-effects include the suppression of new blood cells, which can lead to a severe form of **anaemia**. For this reason, you must have regular blood tests while on this drug. Some doctors also give their patients the B vitamin folic acid, to reduce this side-effect.

Liver damage is also possible with methotrexate, although doctors are finding that liver damage occurs less frequently than they'd anticipated. When used in large doses for the treatment of cancer, this drug causes a high rate of liver damage. But in the dosages used in rheumatoid arthritis about 1 out of every 100 to 200 people taking methotrexate eventually develops some liver damage.

Q How can I find out if I have liver damage?

A   To check for liver damage you need a blood test that assesses a number of the many functions of the liver. This should be done every few weeks. So far as you are concerned, this simply means giving a sample of blood. A problem, though, is that severe liver damage may not show up on this blood test, so after two to three years of taking methotrexate you may want to have a **liver biopsy** to make sure this vital organ is still in tip-top shape. Many GPs, however, do not feel too happy about performing this test for their patients taking methotrexate.

Q **Sounds like I probably shouldn't be drinking alcohol if I'm taking this drug. Right?**

A You're better off if you don't. In fact, you can help to minimize the side-effects of many drugs by avoiding anything more than the occasional drink. It's important to discuss with your doctor how much you actually do drink.

Q **Are there other drugs I should know about?**

A There are others, but they are used much less frequently than those we've mentioned and are not as well studied. They include the immunosuppressive drugs azathioprine, cyclophosphamide and levamisole. These drugs are all in the same general class as methotrexate and act to damp down the immune-system functions that are causing the joint damage in rheumatoid arthritis.

Q **What other questions do I need to ask my doctor about the drugs he or she is prescribing?**

A Any time you're handed a prescription, be prepared to ask questions. What is the exact name of this drug? For what condition or symptoms are you prescribing it? What is the drug supposed to do? How am I supposed to take it? What are the most common side-effects? What are the most serious side-effects? Should I stop the drug if I have side-effects? How long will I be taking this drug? Is there any drug that has the same beneficial effects with fewer side-effects?

Remember also to inquire whether the drug being prescribed could interact with any other drugs you are currently taking. Refresh your doctor's memory on these, if necessary. And don't forget to include any over-the-counter drugs you are taking.

Q **Is it safe to take a new drug that's been on the market only a short time?**

A New and much-lauded drugs have an unfortunate habit of turning out to have unexpected disadvantages. So there's a lot to be said for waiting – even for as long as two or three years – before joining the list of guinea-pigs. This is something you should discuss with your doctor.

Q **If a new and seemingly valuable drug comes out, why should I wait?**

A Because sometimes potentially dangerous side-effects don't show up until a drug has been taken by a lot of people. Of course these drugs are carefully tested before they are issued, but these tests may have been conducted on only a few hundred people – usually reasonably healthy people. Then suddenly, 10,000 people start taking a drug. If a side-effect, even a serious one, occurs in about one person in 200, it might not appear in the preliminary trials. But when a large population of patients take the drug, many cases will present themselves.

SURGERY

Q   **Is surgery ever used to treat arthritis?**
A   Yes. Surgery may be done on a joint to reduce pain and improve function. And, in some cases, it appears to slow the process of joint deterioration, at least for a time.

Q   **What kinds of surgery are done?**
A   Surgery can be done to trim back invading synovial tissue in a joint, to flush particles of debris out of a joint capsule, to smooth out rough cartilage, to improve the angle of impact on an eroding, lopsided knee, to immobilize painful, unstable joints, even to replace a joint that's become unbearably painful and useless.

Q   **How long does a person stay on drug treatment before his or her doctor decides that surgery is needed to alleviate symptoms or restore function to a joint?**
A   There is no definitive answer to this question. It varies from person to person. Let's just say that surgery is rarely the first line of treatment for any kind of arthritis – but it's not necessarily a last resort either. The amount

of time you give drug treatments or steroid injections before you move on to surgical options depends on many variables – which joints are affected, how badly damaged they are, the kind of surgery being contemplated, your general state of health, etc.

Some kinds of surgery prolong the life of a joint enough so that you never require the ultimate in arthritis surgery – total joint replacement. Proper selection of procedure, done for the right reasons and performed by an expert, usually produces good results.

Q How can I determine if I would benefit from surgery?

A If you have a painful joint that is no longer responding to non-surgical treatments such as drugs, rest, splinting or steroid injections, your doctor should refer you to an orthopaedic surgeon, also sometimes called an orthopaedic specialist.

Perhaps, too, you have certain problems in a joint, revealed by x-ray or other imaging technique, which can be improved with surgery. If you have, for example, a severely overgrown synovium, bowed knees or other joint-alignment problems which are wearing down cartilage on one side of a knee, or intermittent pain in a knee that could be due to loose bits of cartilage in the joint capsule, your doctor may refer you to an orthopaedic surgeon for possible surgery.

Q What's the orthopaedic specialist going to do?

A The orthopaedic surgeon will examine your joints, look at your x-rays and probably take some more, and determine if indeed you would benefit from some kind of surgery. Your x-rays, for instance, may show that your hip-joint socket is pitted and that the shock-absorbing cartilage on the head of your thighbone is practically gone.

Q   **Just because this surgeon finds a problem that surgery has been known to improve, does that mean I have to go through with it?**

A   Of course not. No one can force you to accept surgery against your will. But remember that surgeons are busy and are not going to suggest an operation unless they think you are really likely to benefit. Even after being told they could benefit from surgery, however, many people with arthritis take some time to think about it and make up their minds.

    Furthermore, a person may be monitored closely for a while before any definite decisions are made regarding surgery. You see, some hospital rheuma-tologists work in groups which include orthopaedic surgeons. If you're the patient of such a doctor, you may see an orthopaedic surgeon early on for an evaluation; then you might see him or her every year or so for a re-evaluation. Regular consultation with an orthopaedic specialist is one way to determine if or when surgery would be beneficial.

Q   **How can I be sure I will be operated on by the best surgeon and treated in the best hospital?**

A   Anytime you go 'under the knife', and in many cases

under anaesthesia, you want to have the most experienced and qualified surgeon and anaesthetist you can find. Joint surgery, especially total joint replacement, is a highly specialized operation, not just for the surgeon but for the whole surgical team, including the anaesthetist. That means the best place for your operation is a hospital at which your recommended operation is frequently performed, and the best surgeon is one who does that procedure at least several times a week. You should raise this matter with your GP or with the hospital to which you are referred. Don't be shy about asking questions about the qualifications and frequency record of the surgical team you are thinking of entrusting your body to.

One thing you can be reasonably sure about: if you are referred to a major university or teaching hospital, the standard is likely to be of the highest.

Q   **What kinds of surgery are available to people with arthritis?**

A   One of the more common surgical procedures for people with rheumatoid arthritis is **synovectomy**. This is the surgical removal of some of the synovium, the lining of the fluid-filled capsule that surrounds a joint. A normal synovium is paper-thin in width. In a joint affected by rheumatoid arthritis, however, the synovium becomes inflamed and grows wildly, invading the joint capsule and eventually destroying cartilage and bone.

Synovectomy can be done on the knees, wrists and fingers, but not on the hips.

Q   **How does a surgeon work inside a joint capsule? Does the entire joint have to be cut open?**

A   Not necessarily. For a knee joint, a doctor can use **arthroscopic surgery**.

Q   **Arthroscopic surgery? What's that?**

A   Arthroscopic surgery is surgery done on a joint using an **arthroscope**, a flexible viewing tube about the diameter of a pencil. The tube contains optical fibres, a small lens and a light scope. Inserted through a small incision into the joint capsule, an arthroscope provides the surgeon with a view of the joint's inside. The view can be magnified and displayed on a video screen. Instruments that fold down as they are passed through a channel in the arthroscope enable the surgeon to perform some procedures which formerly necessitated opening up the joint. The procedure is usually performed under general anaesthesia, but sometimes a spinal anaesthesia is used. Arthroscopic surgery substantially reduces the time a patient needs to stay in hospital.

Q   **How is synovectomy done using arthroscopic surgery?**

A   The joint capsule is distended by injecting air or fluid; the viewing tube is inserted through a small incision in the knee joint on one side, and a 'cutting sweeper' – a tiny rotary blade attached to a suction tube – is inserted into the knee through two or three other small incisions. Using the viewing scope as a guide, the doctor manoeuvres the cutting sweeper to slice off and suck out some of the overgrown synovial tissue.

Q **How is synovectomy done on other joints?**
A When it's done on smaller joints, such as the wrists or fingers, a synovectomy is done with an incision that exposes the synovium.

Q **Which people most commonly have synovectomies?**
A Synovectomy is normally done only on people with a significant amount of inflamed tissue but little joint damage, and it's done early in the course of the disease. In general, synovectomy is indicated for someone whose inflamed joint has failed to improved with drugs, including steroid injections, but whose x-rays show that the cartilage remains healthy.

Removing the synovium does not cure the underlying disease, but it can prevent a recurrence of inflammation in that joint, sometimes for a few years and sometimes permanently.

Q **What else can be done surgically for arthritis?**
A Arthroscopic debridement is a relatively common procedure, used only on knees. It flushes out of the joint capsule tiny bits of cartilage and bone, along with tissue-eroding enzymes. Any frayed edges of cartilage are removed at the same time.

Arthroscopic debridement is often done on people with osteoarthritis whose x-rays suggest that they have not suffered much joint damage but who are, nevertheless, having a lot of pain that is not relieved by anti-inflammatory drugs or steroid injections. People with knees that lock because loose cartilage bodies are interfering with normal joint action can get excellent results from this procedure. It would not be appropriate for people whose joint is so severely damaged that joint-replacement surgery is obviously indicated.

Q   How well does this procedure work?
A   Sixty to 80 per cent of people who have arthroscopic debridement on a knee have reduced pain for months, sometimes for as long as a year or so. It's not to be expected that this procedure does anything to check the progress of the disease, but it involves minimal risk and recovery is rapid.

Q   Is arthroscopic surgery used for any other kinds of procedures?
A   Yes. It can be used for a variety of joint 'housekeeping and repair' chores, including cartilage and ligament repairs, pinning fractures in a joint and removing scar tissue.

Q   Is arthroscopic surgery risky?
A   Studies show it has an overall complication rate of about one-half of 1 per cent. Risks include infection, nerve or blood-vessel damage and blood clots. As with any surgical procedure, it's best to find a doctor who does this type of surgery regularly.

Q   **Are there any other surgical techniques for the arthritic knee?**

A   Yes. One procedure, called an osteotomy, is performed to correct the angles at which the bones of a joint meet and, thus, to restore normal anatomy to an arthritic joint. It's most often done on knees. A wedge-shaped piece of bone is removed from above or below the joint to correct a bow-leg or knock-knee and distribute the body's weight more evenly across the cartilage of the joint.

   This form of surgery is done mostly on younger active people, especially those with osteoarthritis affecting only one side of a joint – usually as a result of the poor alignment of the joint surfaces. In some cases osteotomy seems to produce a complete answer to the problem, but if it does not, at least there is a reasonable expectation that it will defer more radical surgery for quite some time.

Q   **I've heard that people sometimes have joints fused to stop their pain?**

A   The medical term for bone fusion is **arthrodesis**. In this surgical procedure, two or more bones in a diseased joint are joined together to prevent the joint from moving.

   The precise technique used depends on which joint is being fused, but in most cases cartilage and a surface layer of bone are removed from each bone. The ends of the bones are then placed in close apposition so that they heal together in exactly the same way as a clean fracture would heal. Movement at the site would tend to prevent this from happening, so the bones may need to be fastened in position with plates, rods or screws to immobilize the area while the bones grow together. Sometimes a joint, such as a knee, may need to be immobilized for a time with pins inserted through the skin into the joint, to keep the joint from moving when body weight is applied. It can take up to six months for a fused joint to heal.

Q   **In what circumstances is this procedure done?**

A   Fusion is done when no other better options, such as joint replacement, are available, and treatments such as steroid injections have failed. Fusing a joint is a fairly desperate expedient and is done as a last resort. The real point of doing it is that it generally does eliminate pain, and it can restore some function to a joint which has previously been useless. But, of course, it also reduces joint mobility to zero, and this can be seriously disabling. If it's done on an ankle or knee, for instance, it affects the patient's gait. It's most likely to be done on wrists or ankles – there are no good replacement parts for these complicated joints – but it can also be done, when necessary, on knees, hips, ankles and fingers.

Q   **Do people with arthritis ever have bones removed? What's this procedure and when is it done?**

A   Removing anything in surgery is called a resection. In the case of bones, resection involves removal of part or all of a damaged bone to help realign a joint which is permanently and painfully dislocated.

Resection can be done on any small joint, but it's done most frequently in the feet when damaged bones make walking painful in spite of treatment with drugs, steroid injections or orthopaedic shoe inserts. Parts of the metatarsal bones, the long bones that extend from the ankles to the toes, are most likely to be removed.

A foot may be wider and flatter after this operation, but the patient can still walk on it, often without pain. Resection may also be done to certain sections of the wrist or thumb.

Q You've mentioned joint replacement several times. What is it?

A Joint-replacement surgery is a procedure to replace all or part of a joint – that is, the joining bones. A total-joint replacement, of course, replaces the whole joint.

Joint-replacement surgery is done when cartilage and underlying bone in a joint are so eroded and damaged that the joint hurts most of the time and the pain is severely limiting the person's activity.

Even though joint replacement often relieves pain and restores some function to joints, it's considered a last resort – an option to consider when drugs, steroid injections, rest and even less drastic forms of surgery have failed.

Q If it works so well, why would it be considered a last resort?

A First, this is major surgery involving the removal of a substantial part of the body. Secondly, however ingenious and well-designed, artificial joints do have a limited life span, usually because they come loose in the bones to which they are fixed, or even break. That life span is slowly increasing, though, thanks to better surgical techniques and more resilient replacement materials. Progress is slow because a new design of joint has to be tested for at least the life-span of prior designs before it can be shown to be superior.

Q   **How long can I expect my artificial joint to last?**

A   This varies from person to person, depending on age, activity level and weight, among other things. The first generation of hip-joint replacements (those put in from 1968 to 1974) were plagued by problems. Infection rates were high, and loosening and breakage were not uncommon. Now the track record is much better. Studies show that 9 out of 10 people who get a hip replacement at age 60 still have a functioning hip 10 years later. Fifteen years later, 80 to 85 per cent still have a well-functioning hip.

Artificial hips that are placed in younger people actually have a shorter life span. Among people aged 50 to 60, only 80 per cent still have a functioning hip joint 10 years after it's first installed. This is because these prosthetic joints are simply worn out by these more active people. This is why some surgeons are reluctant to undertake hip joint replacement in patients under the age of 60.

Artificial knees, too, encountered problems early on, but as today's artificial knee-joint design sticks closely to the structure of an actual knee joint, using both plastic and metal to form a joint that not only bends but also slightly twists and turns, like the real thing, they appear to have a life span as good as or slightly better than artificial hips. Nine out of 10 people who get a knee replacement at the age of 60 still have a functioning knee 10 years later.

Q **What about people younger than age 50? Do they ever get artificial joints?**

A If at all possible, joint replacement is avoided in people younger than 50. This may not be possible if someone has severe rheumatoid arthritis or osteoarthritis and needs this operation to be able to function. In this case, the surgeon would have to be quite frank about the probability that, at some time in the future, the operation might have to be done again – a procedure called a **revision**.

Q **Could you explain what a revision entails?**

A A revision is an operation to refix or replace an artificial joint that has loosened, broken or become infected. Unfortunately, a revision does not usually last as long as the original joint replacement. Most surgeons would expect a revision to last for at least five years, however. As for further revisions, this is something surgeons view with a marked lack of enthusiasm. It is a law of diminishing returns: the more often you repeat the procedure the shorter becomes the expected life span of the joint.

Revision requires at least as much surgical skill as the original joint replacement, perhaps more, if the surgeon has to contend with bone loss from the loosened prosthesis. Here again, specialists emphasize, your best results should come from a surgeon who has a considerable experience of this sort of surgery.

Q   **Which joints are most likely to be replaced?**
A   Hip joints, without any question. This is now one of the most commonly performed major operations. Not all hip replacements are done because of arthritis, however. Fractures of the neck of the femur are very common in elderly women as a result of osteoporosis, and this often leads to a loss of the blood supply to, and degeneration of, the ball of the femur. In this event joint replacement is often the best option.

Knee-joint replacement, formerly rare, is now becoming increasingly common, too, as better designs become available. Joint-replacement surgery can also be done on fingers and, much less frequently (because the results aren't all that good), on shoulders and elbows.

Q   **What exactly is done in joint-replacement surgery?**
A   Any kind of joint replacement – whether it's a hip, knee or even a finger – is a complicated, technically-demanding procedure that requires a full team of experienced orthopaedic surgeons, assistants and operating theatre staff. Special and meticulous precautions are necessary to avoid infection.

For a hip replacement, done under general anaesthesia, the surgeon makes a large incision on the side of the hip and pushes or cuts through the surrounding muscles to expose the hip joint. The joint is then dislocated, so that the ball-shaped head of the femur is popped out of its socket in the pelvis (the acetabulum). Next the surgeon saws off the head of the femur, then uses an instrument called a reamer to make the acetabulum large enough to hold the cup-shaped artificial socket. Then the artificial socket is inserted.

The surgeon now uses a coarse file to ream out the open hollow cut end of the shaft of the femur, and inserts the stem of the ball part of the artificial joint into the bone. A grouting-type cement may or may not be used to hold the stem in place. Special cements which will bond wet bone to cold metal and yet will not excite a tissue reaction must be used. Once this part of the prosthetic joint is secure, the surgeon manipulates the leg so that the ball slips into the socket. Where necessary, muscles are then reattached to bones with wires or strong collagen stitches. Other muscles and tendons are replaced and repaired, and finally the incision is closed.

Q   **And how is this surgery done for knees?**

A   With knees, also done under general anaesthesia, the surgeon usually makes one long incision on the front of the joint. He or she cuts through the joint capsule and synovium, then pushes aside the kneecap (patella) to get at the joint.

Special surgical tools are used to measure the joint carefully and to cut, shape and drill both the femur and the tibia (the larger lower leg bone) so that they can accept the artificial joint. Both are screwed into place and are often cemented.

The bottom half of the knee joint is a metal plate with a slight depression in its centre. The top half is a metal cap that fits over this rounded bone. The metal cap rests in the bottom plate. Part of the back of the kneecap is cut away to give a flat surface, and is then drilled to accept the kneecap part of the joint.

Since the same ligaments that hold a natural knee joint in place are needed to maintain an artificial knee joint, only knees with intact or surgically repaired ligaments are acceptable for joint-replacement surgery.

Q   What about fingers?

A   Done before surrounding support tissues, such as tendons, have deteriorated, joint-replacement surgery of fingers can usually restore pain-free motion. Usually it's only the largest knuckles that are replaced, and then only in people with rheumatoid arthritis.

Q   Do people with osteoarthritis ever have finger joint-replacement surgery?

A   People with osteoarthritis may have bone-spur bumps around their knuckles which make their joints appear swollen, but they seldom lose the ability to use their hands, so they rarely require surgery.

Q   Is it better to have hand surgery done as soon as possible?

A   That depends. It is true that decisions to operate on hands are made differently from decisions to operate on hips or knees. One risk is that if surgery is delayed there is a possibility of tendon rupture before the operation. The results are much better if tendons remain intact and fully functional at the time of surgery. It's not possible, however, to tell whether tendon rupture is imminent, so some surgical specialists have what they call 'the six-month rule'. If a patient has had pain in the hands or wrists for six months and it hasn't responded to drugs or steroid injections, the risk of tendon rupture rises steeply. So these surgeons will usually want to operate.

Q   What material is used for a finger joint?

A   Replacement finger joints are made out of a silicone-rubber material. They are one piece, with a stem on either end and a flexible hinged piece in the middle. The stems insert into the bones of the finger, but are not fixed in place. In fact, they move slightly in and out as you bend your fingers.

Q   What happens during this operation?

A   This operation can take several hours, depending on how many joints are replaced and on what else is done to the hand. A regional anaesthesia is used to numb part of the arm as well as the hand and fingers. An incision is made to expose the joint; the ends of the two diseased bones in the joint are cut away, taking the diseased cartilage with them. The artificial joint is then inserted, and the tissue and underlying skin are sewn up. If you have this operation, your knuckles will be bandaged and your arm will be held upward in a sling to minimize swelling. You won't be able to use your hands at all for about four days, and you'll have limited use for about six to eight weeks, while you undergo extensive physiotherapy. You can expect to regain full normal use of your hands in two to three months.

Q **Is cement always used to hold a joint replacement in place?**

A There are some new replacement joints on the market which don't need to be cemented into the bones. These joints have a fibre mesh or beaded surface that invites bone to grow into the artificial joint and, so, secure it. Cemented joints tend to loosen as tissue grows between the cement and the bone. It's thought that the new fibre-mesh joints will be less likely than cemented joints to loosen over time.

Q **So how long will they last?**

A No one knows for sure yet just how long these new non-cemented joints will last. Studies so far seem to show that on the cup, or socket, side of a hip joint, the non-cemented component is very effective. There have been no high rates of early failure and no significant problems at 5 or 10 years.

On the stem side, however, where loosening forces are much stronger, results have been mixed. In the short term, one or two years after surgery, the non-cemented joint tends to fare worse than the cemented. This does not necessarily mean that they are coming dangerously loose, but patients are more likely to have thigh pain than they would with a cemented joint.

Results of studies have led many doctors to use a non-cemented socket in most of their hip-joint replacements, no matter what a person's age, and often a non-cemented stem, or ball joint, in people younger than age 65. The results with the cemented joint aren't as good in younger, more active, people. So there is a tendency to go for the newer non-cemented joints in a younger person with good bone quality, hoping for effective bone growth into the replacement joint so as to give a more stable long-term result.

Q **What about knees? Are they cemented?**
A Non-cemented knees have not worked as well as hips, and many doctors have stopped using them, at least for now.

Q **I'm worried that a surgeon might suggest an unnecessary operation, perhaps just to practise or to try out a new idea. Do I need to worry about having unnecessary surgery for arthritis?**
A Absolutely not. These days surgeons are so busy that they get all the practice they need on people who really need surgery. And no surgeon is going to try out a new and experimental procedure without your full informed consent. This is a legal requirement.

If you are still worried, you can always ask for a second opinion, perhaps from a rheumatologist, who can check to make sure you've given all non-surgical alternatives a fair try. Or you might even ask to see another surgeon who will give you an unbiased opinion. Orthopaedic surgeons see patients every day for consultations, and only a proportion of these patients end up in theatre. And remember, no matter what your doctor or surgeon tells you, it's up to you to decide whether or not to have the operation. Many times, with arthritis, this is a decision you can sit on for a while, because joint deterioration tends to be slow, albeit steady. Sometimes, however, your operation will turn out better if it's done promptly. This would be the case, for instance, if you had inflamed tendons that could rupture.

Q Any other questions I need to ask?

A Often, several kinds of surgical procedures are used together to repair a joint, especially a complicated joint like a wrist. So ask exactly what procedures the doctor is recommending and why. Find out, too, what you can expect as a result of the operation. Reduced pain? More strength in your hand? Increased mobility? Decreased mobility? Are you going to be able to walk? Play tennis? Open a jar? Scratch your back? Pick up a pound coin? And how long should these results last?

Ask, too, how long your recovery may take and what it entails. Major orthopaedic surgery is inevitably followed by physical rehabilitation, and you want to make sure you're up to the challenge.

Q **Anything else I need to know?**

A If you're having joint-replacement surgery, you should get into the best possible state of health you can beforehand. If you have any kind of infection, even an aching tooth, you should have it treated before your operation. Otherwise, there's a risk that the infection could get to your new joint.

If you're overweight, your doctor will want you to lose some pounds before you have hip or knee joint-replacement surgery. That's because extra weight puts stress on a joint and could make it heal slower and loosen sooner.

Good muscle tone is important, too, so if you're able to do so, continue your exercise programme.

If you're taking certain drugs for your arthritis, you may need to discontinue them for a week or two before your operation. Be sure to talk to your doctor and surgeon about this. Anti-inflammatory drugs and fish-oil capsules can increase the amount of time it takes for your blood to clot, making bleeding more of a problem. Even aspirin can have a significant effect on blood clotting. And immunosuppressive drugs for rheumatoid arthritis, such as methotrexate, may prevent a surgical wound from healing and, therefore, may have to be stopped for a time.

CHAPTER FOUR

ALTERNATIVE SOURCES
OF HELP

Q   **In addition to drugs and surgery, are there other kinds
    of help for arthritis?**

A   Yes, many. People with arthritis may be prescribed one
    or more of a great range of treatments to ease their
    aches and pains. Medical care for arthritis often includes
    physiotherapy, exercise classes, occupational therapy
    and the use of joint-protecting splints, pain-easing
    massage, whirlpools, paraffin wax dips, heat and cold
    treatments, and other hands-on therapies. Several good
    studies now show that regular exercise can ease pain
    and improve joint mobility in just about everyone with
    arthritis, no matter their age or how long they've had
    arthritis. We'll talk more about these studies and how
    to find an exercise programme that suits you a little
    later in this chapter.

Q   **What about treatments performed by non-medical
    practitioners?**

A   Many people with arthritis seek alternative treatments,
    such as **acupuncture**, herbal remedies, Swedish massage

or special diets. In fact, people with arthritis spend many millions of pounds a year on a long, long list of alternative or scientifically unproven remedies, from copper bracelets to **DMSO (dimethyl sulphoxide)** to mussel extracts. Since these remedies have never been *proven*, at least not by the kind of scientific standards most doctors consider essential, it's up to you to decide whether a particular remedy is worth trying and what its possible risks are. In this chapter we'll tell you the kinds of questions you need to ask to evaluate a non-traditional remedy.

Q **Aren't there some treatments that involve diet and nutrition?**

A Yes. Some of these include dietary changes. In fact, there is some intriguing evidence that dietary additions or deletions can help some people with arthritis, either by eliminating a symptom-producing food or by altering the body's inflammatory response. If you're interested in making dietary changes, we'll tell you how to get started safely.

Q **Aren't there treatments that really are experimental – where I become in effect a guinea pig?**

A Some people with arthritis do indeed decide to become medical guinea pigs. They enrol in research studies, called clinical trials, which examine a treatment that may show promise but that has not been proven to work. Some of these studies are organized by hospital specialists anxious to improve the effectiveness of the treatment they can offer. Other studies are funded by drug companies, and are usually conducted in conjunction with hospital specialists.

EXERCISE

Q   **Well, it certainly seems I should have a lot of information before I start any new treatment scheme. Can you tell me more?**

A   Let's start with exercise, which gets top ratings from patients and doctors alike when it comes to relieving arthritis symptoms. In one major survey, the authors amassed the answers of more than 1,000 people with arthritis. An overwhelming majority of participants said they exercise regularly because of their arthritis, and fully 95 per cent said it helped. A small number said they found exercise too painful to pursue. And 17 per cent had been hurt at least once by inappropriate or overzealous physical activity – a good reason to get guidance before you begin.

Q   **How does exercise help arthritis?**

A   For both rheumatoid arthritis and osteoarthritis, a properly designed, faithfully followed exercise programme can get you moving and keep you moving. It can improve muscle strength, build stamina and allow joints to move better, with less pain and swelling. It may also allow some people to cut back on anti-inflammatory drugs. And it can replace feelings of fatigue and depression with new energy and optimism.

Q **How can I find a properly designed exercise pro-gramme?**

A Start with the doctor who is treating your arthritis. Ask for a referral to a physiotherapist – one who treats people with arthritis. Working in conjunction with your doctor, the physiotherapist can set up a daily exercise programme to keep your joints as mobile and healthy as possible, or to help you recover from joint surgery. If you need special equipment to exercise – a splint, cane or special shoes – the physiotherapy department can also provide these.

A physiotherapist is also likely to be involved in some of the more pleasant treatments associated with arthritis – whirlpool baths, hot-wax treatments for hands, and massage.

Q **What kinds of exercise can people with arthritis do? And what kinds should they avoid?**

A People with arthritis should avoid pounding, bouncy or jerky exercises, such as high-impact aerobics, racket sports or running. But most can safely do many things: walking, bicycling, swimming, yoga, even in some cases, moderate weight lifting. The key is to get your doctor's approval and proper instruction before you start on any of these activities, so you don't suffer start-up injuries that put you permanently on the sidelines.

Many people do range-of-motion exercises regularly to keep their joints flexible. These exercises attempt to take each joint in the body through its full range. A physiotherapist can teach you these exercises.

HEAT AND COLD

Q   I love whirlpool baths and hot tubs. Do they do anything to help my arthritis?

A   Many people with arthritis find that settling into a hot tub soothes every joint in their body. Some use that buoyant, muscle-relaxing opportunity to do their range-of-motion exercises. Others use the whirlpool jets to give themselves a water massage. Pleasant as these soaks are, however, most people with arthritis say they offer only temporary relief and do not have any real long-term value.

Q   What about other forms of heat? What do they do?

A   Heating pads, electric blankets, even dipping the hands in hot paraffin wax can all ease the stiffness and pain in aching joints, at least temporarily. Again, it's the heat, which increases blood flow to the area, that does the trick. In fact, many people with arthritis loosen up their stiff joints a bit with some form of heat prior to exercising.

Q   I've often heard that applying cold helps. Does it?

A   Cold, which reduces blood flow to an area, seems to work well to reduce pain and is usually your best choice for a hot, inflamed joint or a joint or muscle that's been overworked.

Q   Are there any risks with heat or cold treatments?

A   Heat is not always appropriate and can even aggravate

some symptoms. Your best bet is to learn how to use both heat and cold with the guidance of a physiotherapist.

For instance, experts say you should not apply heat to one area for more than 20 to 30 minutes. And don't apply cold to one area for more than 10 to 20 minutes. Don't use heat or cold if you have poor circulation or poor sensation in the area. Don't use heat on a joint that's just been rubbed with a heat-producing analgesic cream, because the combination can damage your skin.

Q   **What is a deep heat treatment?**
A   **Deep heat** therapy uses tissue-penetrating ultrasound waves to heat up small areas of the body. In fact, this is the only heat treatment that can penetrate beyond the surface layers of the skin to a joint. In one survey, 81 per cent of the people who tried ultrasound said it helped ease their pain and stiffness. Like other heat treatments, though, ultrasound is not always appropriate and may aggravate inflamed joints. This treatment is given by a qualified physiotherapist.

Q   **How about massage? Does it help?**
A   Massage can help relax tense muscles and improve circulation, and certain types of massage can help move fluid out of a swollen limb. But massage directly applied to a painful, inflamed joint can be harmful. If you're interested in getting a massage, ask your doctor or physiotherapist for a referral to a massage therapist who works regularly with people with arthritis.

OCCUPATIONAL THERAPIST

Q   **What about health-care professionals like occupational therapists? Can they help?**

A   An occupational therapist – whose primary goal is to restore a degree of functioning – can show you how to protect your joints, carry on the normal activities of life in the best ways possible, and recommend special aids that make it easier to do things such as open a jar, reach a high object, or even turn a steering wheel in a car.

An occupational therapist can also devise splints that help keep joints in normal positions, and so prevent permanent joint deformities which are hard to correct by reconstructive surgery.

Q   **You've mentioned splints before. What exactly does a splint do?**

A   A splint – usually made of plastic which can be heated slightly then moulded around a wrist or finger – can prevent weak muscles from being stretched and can support joints by substituting for weak muscles. It can be used to keep an inflamed joint in its least painful position and reduce the possibility of a permanent deformity.

Some people wear wrist splints to bed, for instance, so that their wrists don't get bent into painful positions during the night. Others may wear them while using their hands for repetitive motions.

These days, though, doctors don't like to keep joints totally immobilized for too long for fear they'll become

too weak and stiff to move. You may get a recommendation to remove your splint daily and put your joint
through range-of-motion exercises.

CHIROPRACTOR

Q **What about chiropractors? How are they trained?
Can they help someone with arthritis?**

A A chiropractor is a non-medical practitioner who may
or may not have had formal training and registration.
Members of the British Chiropractic Association must
have a BSc degree in chiropractic and have completed a
one-year course at an established clinic.

Chiropractic is based on the principle that the spinal
column is central to a person's entire sense of wellbeing.
The treatments provided involve spinal manipulation, or
adjustments, in which the chiropractor pushes on the
vertebrae to reposition alleged displacements.

Since chiropractors are concerned with the structure
of the body, they are required to study anatomy,
physiology, neurophysiology, biomechanics and kinesi-
ology. This training, as well as the use of certain diagnostic procedures, permits chiropractors to consider
the body's entire neuro-musculoskeletal system when
making a diagnosis.

Studies have shown that chiropractic adjustments
may offer people with arthritis some temporary relief.
This may be in the form of increased mobility in a stiff-
ened spine. But overall, there is little evidence that

chiropractors can provide substantial help for people with arthritis. A sizable percentage of people have found that they feel worse after they have seen a chiropractor.

Forceful mobilization is not what arthritic sufferers need, especially during phases of acute inflammation. If you are having chiropractic treatment be sure to tell your chiropractor about any change in your symptoms since his or her initial evaluation of you. You should also tell your chiropractor if you feel you're having a flare-up. In fairness, it must be said that chiropractors who find x-ray and other evidence of any bone or joint disease, including arthritis, will wish to refer patients to orthodox doctors.

PSYCHOTHERAPIST

Q   **What if I'm having trouble coping with my illness? Whom can I see then?**

A   A psychotherapist may be able to help you adjust to your illness and limitations, and to help you free up your mental energies so you can get on with your life. Some psychotherapists can also teach techniques such as biofeedback and progressive relaxation, which studies have shown do reduce pain and stress, so that you require less medication, sleep better and feel more in control.

Shop for a psychotherapist as you would for any health-care professional. Ask the doctor treating your arthritis for a referral, and ask other people with arthritis. Check the Yellow Pages and phone in to try to find a listed psychotherapist who treats people with arthritis or other chronic illnesses.

Have a get-acquainted visit, and, based on your impressions from that first visit, decide if this psychotherapist might be of some help.

DIETITIAN

Q You mentioned earlier that nutrition and dietary changes may help some people with arthritis. What kind of health-care professional would I see for that?

A A registered dietitian can help you make dietary changes.

If you need to lose weight to take a load off aching knees, for instance, a dietitian can help you to devise a weight-loss programme that allows you to lose weight sensibly and gradually, without compromising good nutrition. He or she can also help you to select vitamin and mineral supplements when appropriate, and steer you through the maze of dietary treatments for arthritis, which we'll discuss shortly.

Q What is a dietitian?

A A dietitian is a qualified health professional who has undertaken formal study and obtained a registrable qualification in dietetics – the whole science of food, food preparation, requirements in health and disease, food intake and nutrition. Dietitians have university degrees in the subject and have undergone prescribed work in recognized institutions.

Q   **How can I get in touch with a dietitian?**

A   If your doctor or hospital specialist thinks that a dietitian would help, you can be referred. Most hospitals have a dietitian on staff. Don't expect miracle cures from a dietitian, however, and don't expect a dietitian to show much sympathy with the dietetic theories put forward by many alternative practitioners.

Q   **Are there any alternative treatments I should avoid?**

A   It all depends. It's always wise to approach any new treatment – even popular arthritis drugs – with extreme scepticism. If you must go in for alternative treatments, find a practitioner with lots of experience and, if you're using a treatment at home, make sure you really do know how to do it and that you understand its potential hazards. Even something as simple as a heating pad can do harm if used in the wrong way.

Ask questions to determine if the treatment is appropriate and helpful for your condition. Are there any studies published which show its effectiveness for arthritis? What has been the practitioner's experience in using the treatment for arthritis? Can you talk with other arthritis patients who have used the treatment? Do you feel better after you've had a treatment?

DIET

Q   I've heard that certain foods can cause arthritis, or at least make it worse. Is that true?

A   Only one type of arthritis, gout, has been definitely connected with diet. Foods high in **purines** – protein compounds found in anchovies, organ meats and mushrooms, among other foods – can aggravate the condition by elevating body levels of uric acid. The uric acid builds up to high levels in synovial fluid and forms joint-irritating crystals.

Some intriguing research findings, however, do suggest that food plays a role in other types of arthritis as well, or at least in some sorts of joint inflammation which may resemble arthritis. Food may provoke joint inflammation in two ways, which we'll detail a bit later. Meanwhile, here are some suggested links between food and arthritis.

In a small number of sensitive people, certain foods may provoke an allergic inflammatory reaction in joint tissue, just as it might cause hives or asthma in other sensitive people. Such people may find that eliminating these foods from their diet helps relieve joint inflammation.

The kinds of fat a person eats seem to influence the body's inflammatory response, too. Researchers believe that some fats promote the manufacture of inflammation-producing biochemicals known as prostaglandins, while other fats, such as fish oil, interfere with the manufacture of these substances. Indeed, some studies show that certain fatty acids can be helpful to people with rheumatoid arthritis.

Q **What kinds of studies have been done on food allergies and arthritis? What do they show?**

A The food-arthritis link is highly controversial, and most doctors believe there are not enough hard facts (that is, good controlled clinical studies) to say for sure that food sensitivities can *cause* arthritis, especially when it comes to rheumatoid arthritis. You may recall from Chapter 2 that the cause of rheumatoid arthritis remains unknown, although many suspect it starts with exposure to something that alters immune response – perhaps a virus or bacterium.

Research into the food-arthritis link includes single-case studies (in which a doctor looks at one patient), a few animal studies and a few dietary-restriction studies in which people with rheumatoid arthritis tried a certain kind of diet to see if their symptoms improved.

Several of the single-case studies suggest that a small number of people do indeed get flare-ups of arthritis when they eat certain foods.

Q **What more can you tell me about these case studies?**

A You must appreciate that the scientific work done on this is very limited. When patients were given various foods disguised in capsules so that they did not know what they were taking, three out of 15 experienced arthritis symptoms. One reacted to milk, another to shrimp, and the third to **nitrates**, a common food preservative.

One person tested was a 52-year-old woman who insisted her arthritis was caused by meat, milk and beans. She agreed to go on an extremely restricted diet for several weeks and ate nothing except a liquid diet, free from these ingredients. The result was that she was not bothered by stiff joints during this time.

Then, in what's called a double-blind, placebo-controlled test, she was given the foods she claimed were causing her symptoms. In this tightly controlled test, neither she nor the people giving her the foods knew what foods she was receiving. The foods, in powdered form, were in opaque capsules. And not all the capsules contained a food she claimed were causing her symptoms. Some were placebos – harmless sugar pills.

At the end of this study, it was clear that the culprit was milk. When the woman ate capsules of powdered milk, her morning stiffness and tender, swollen joints returned. Symptoms were worst within 24 to 48 hours after ingesting the milk, and subsided within three days.

Q **Are there other foods that cause symptoms of arthritis?**

A In individual case reports by other researchers, cheese, corn, wheat and other foods have been associated with RA-like symptoms.

Q **What about animal studies?**

A In a study with rabbits, rheumatoid-like inflammation of the synovium was induced simply by substituting cow's milk for water in the diet.

Q   **And dietary-restriction studies?**

A   Several studies have looked at all sorts of dietary restrictions. The results of these studies have been mixed. It does rather seem that arbitrarily restricted diets often miss the point. People with a particular sensitivity to one food substance should not have to go on rigid diets which cut out a great many perfectly safe ingredients. One American study, for instance, tested a popular arthritis diet, called the Dong diet after its inventor Dr Collin H. Dong. The diet eliminated red meat, additives, preservatives, fruit, dairy products, herbs, spices and alcohol. This highly restrictive diet certainly improved symptoms in a few people, but seemed to work no better than a diet that arbitrarily eliminated foods such as sour cream, turkey, bananas and cornflakes, while allowing red meat and white wine. A few people did seem to exhibit reduced joint swelling on the Dong diet, but when some of these people were later tested individually, they were found to be sensitive to certain foods.

Q   **I've heard that a vegetarian diet can help people with arthritis. Is this true?**

A   Yes, it has been noted that people with rheumatoid arthritis do better on a vegetarian diet. However, only one study, by researcher Lars Skoldstam of the Sundvall Hospital in Sundvall, Sweden, has looked at the effects of a vegetarian diet on rheumatoid arthritis. In that study, 60 per cent of the people with rheumatoid arthritis who followed a **vegan diet** – which excludes dairy products as well as meat – said they felt better on the diet. We should mention, too, that the diet also excluded or limited the use of refined sugar, corn, flour, salt, strong spices, alcohol, tea and coffee.

This researcher didn't claim to know how the diet worked, but it's possible it eliminated some of the foods to which people with rheumatoid arthritis were sensitive.

Q **What about not eating at all?**

A Yes, **fasting** – going without food – does seem to relieve symptoms in people with rheumatoid arthritis, according to several studies. Unfortunately, in most cases, the relief disappears soon after the fast is broken.

In one Swedish study, eight out of 10 people said they felt much better while fasting. For 11 days they had nothing but vegetarian broths, juices made from vegetables or berries and herbal teas every two or three hours. We should mention, however, that two members of the group grew worse.

Q **What is it about fasting that relieves symptoms of arthritis in some people?**

A Fasting has a modulating effect on the immune system, according to some researchers. It slows the action of certain enzymes and blocks the production of biochemicals that cause inflammation.

Other researchers point out that fasting eliminates any symptom-causing foods. Some think it may improve conditions in the bowel, at least temporarily. Some forms of inflammatory arthritis have been associated with inflammatory bowel disease.

If you're in good health and not taking drugs, most doctors agree that one to three days of fasting won't hurt you. But for most people with RA this would not be good advice. They're underweight and may even be malnourished. For them, the risks of fasting could offset its short-term benefits.

Q **So, for some people, food might be a factor in joint pain. But what's the mechanism behind it?**

A It has to do with the body's immune system. In cases in which a food seems to be causing an allergic reaction, researchers speculate that somehow a person's intestinal wall becomes permeable – meaning it allows passage of things that would normally be blocked. This may be due to inflammation, bacterial overgrowth, an allergic tendency or even taking anti-inflammatory drugs. The intestinal wall allows large molecules of a food – perhaps some of those found in milk, for instance – that it can't normally absorb, to pass through the intestinal membrane and into the bloodstream. There, the large molecules are treated by the body's immune system as though they were harmful invaders.

In response to these molecules (called antigens), the body's immune cells develop antibodies. These antibodies can latch onto the antigen as it's absorbed through the gut, and become larger objects called circulating immune complexes, which go around in the body's bloodstream until they can find a good place to be deposited. Circulating immune complexes may stick to blood-vessel walls, where they cause hives and vasculitis. Or a very common place for them to go is into the joints, especially if the joint is already damaged by an arthritic flare-up. In the joint, the immune complexes lie on the synovium. There, they attract large scavenging phagocytes – cells called macrophages – which gobble up the immune complexes and, in the process, damage the joint tissue as well, causing localized inflammation.

It's also possible for a food antigen to travel alone to a joint, and there be attacked by antibodies that are on the surface of **mast cells** in the synovium. When this happens, the mast cells detonate like microscopic bombs, releasing a spray of inflammatory biochemicals – such as histamine, leukotrienes and prostaglandins – into your joint, destroying the antigen and perhaps damaging joint cells as well.

Mast cells are known to play a large part in allergic reactions, especially in such conditions as hay fever and asthma. They may also be significantly involved in the causation of arthritis. Abnormally attractive mast cell receptors for antibodies can occur as a result of a genetic mutation. It has recently been found that certain of these receptors which seem to encourage antibody adhesion are present in people with the hereditary tendency to allergy (known as atopy). So far, atopy seems relevant only to asthma, hay fever and eczema, but the significance of this may be more widespread than we think.

Q   **What percentage of people with rheumatoid arthritis have symptoms aggravated by food?**

A   There is no official figure, but those who know most about the subject suggest that it is 5 per cent or less. Some doctors claim, without hard evidence to prove it, that the figure may be as high as 30 per cent.

It seems that people whose arthritis is affected by food do not show some of the other classic symptoms of rheumatoid arthritis, such as joint deterioration and the presence of rheumatoid factor in the blood. At least one expert has termed food-aggravated arthritis *allergic arthritis* to distinguish it from rheumatoid arthritis.

Q   **Do people with rheumatoid arthritis pain have many allergic symptoms, such as skin or nasal allergies?**

A   Research seems to indicate that they do not. There is no evidence that general allergic disease is any more common in people with rheumatoid arthritis than it is in the general population. Also, people with allergies are no more prone to RA than anyone else. This suggests that either atopy is not involved in the causation of RA or that the form of food allergy involved in RA is basically different from those in the more common allergic conditions such as hay fever, asthma and eczema.

Q   **What foods are most likely to cause symptoms of arthritis?**

A   As we said earlier, research is scant, but in several studies milk or cheese was found to cause symptoms. In fact, researchers in Switzerland have found changes in the immune system of people who appear to be milk-sensitive. These same researchers tested two people who appeared to be highly sensitive to whole milk and found they reacted to a specific protein in milk. Corn, shrimp, nitrates, beef and wheat have also been implicated in some cases.

   Some researchers believe, too, that a certain family of vegetables, called **nightshades**, can cause symptoms of joint inflammation for some people.

Q   **What are nightshades?**

A   Nightshades are the *solanaceous* botanical family which includes potatoes, eggplants, tomatoes and peppers (red and green bell peppers, chili peppers and paprika, but not black pepper). This group also includes tobacco and some other very toxic plants, such as belladonna (called *deadly nightshade*), henbane, mandrake and jimsonweed.

   Even the edible members of this family have long been viewed with suspicion. In the early 1800s, most people believed that raw tomatoes could kill you.

Q   **But can they cause arthritis?**

A   It seems that a small percentage of arthritis sufferers are nightshade-sensitive and will benefit from the elimination of all foods containing these vegetables from their diets. The American scientist who came up with the no-nightshades diet, Norman F. Childers, believes a number of substances that are found in all these plants cause symptoms, including **solanine**. Solanine is a known toxin, and it has been associated with joint inflammation in animals. However, most doctors believe you don't get enough of it in any of these foods to do you harm.

Dr Childers says he has surveyed thousands of people with arthritis who tried his no-nightshade diet, and says about 70 per cent found some relief on this diet.

Q **If I wanted to try this diet, what would I do?**
A You should learn how to read food packaging labels. Potato starch and tomato flakes or paste are found in many foods. Also, you should avoid tobacco – for many reasons, not just to comply with this diet.

Quite a few people avoid one food or another. Their collective list of foods to avoid is impressive. It includes red meat, sugar, fats, salt, caffeine, nightshades, alcohol, junk foods, starches (such as wheat), citrus fruit, pork, smoked or processed meats and dairy products. It would be severely limiting, probably impracticable, to try to avoid all these foods in order to eliminate only one or a few. The problem is to decide which ones are out of bounds for you. This may take some doing.

Q   **How can I determine which foods, if any, are causing my symptoms?**

A   One way is to start keeping a journal in which you record everything you eat and in which you also record and rate your joint pain and any swelling. If your symptoms vary from day to day, keeping a food journal might help you to pinpoint troublesome foods.

Another way is to eliminate all forms of the one suspected food from your diet for about two months, then add it back to your diet and see if your symptoms flare up. Don't try to eliminate more than one food at a time.

Some foods, especially those you eat all the time or that are found in many different foods (wheat, for instance), can be difficult to connect with symptoms.

ALLERGIST

Q   **You mean that I may not be able to work out which food I eat frequently is causing my symptoms?**

A   Yes. You may find you need the help of an allergist who treats people with food sensitivities. There are very few allergists practising in Britain, so most allergic problems are handled by other specialists such as GPs, chest specialists, dermatologists and so on. A few immunologists have taken a special interest in food allergy and food intolerance.

One major problem in this context is that there are plenty of people around who *call* themselves allergists but who actually practise some of the more extreme alternative therapies. Few of these people have even an elementary knowledge of the highly complex subject of immunology, and some of them don't even appear to understand what allergy really is.

You have to be careful if you are looking for a genuine allergist. Do make sure that your selected advisor is either medically qualified and has had further training in allergic studies or is a trained biological scientist with a knowledge of modern immunology.

Q **What can an allergist do to help?**

A An allergist can devise a diet which allows you to avoid the offending food substance. Doctors use different sorts of diets. Some use a diet of foods so seldom eaten that someone is unlikely to have developed allergies to them. After a period of time on this diet – a week, perhaps – you'll be asked to reintroduce a specific food and see if your symptoms worsen. If they do worsen, you may want to continue to avoid that food.

Q **You said earlier that fats in my diet can influence my body's inflammatory response. How so?**

A The type of fat you eat helps to determine, at least to some extent, your body's manufacture of hormone-like biochemicals called eicosanoids. These include prostaglandins, thromboxanes and leukotrienes. Some prostaglandins promote inflammation; others control inflammation. The fatty acids in foods are the precursors, or building blocks, for a class of prostaglandins.

Your body takes the fatty acids you eat and, through a series of metabolic steps, assembles them into either pro-inflammatory or anti-inflammatory prostaglandins.

Q   **What kinds of fats are pro-inflammatory?**

A   Most vegetable oils – safflower, sunflower, corn, sesame and soy oil – are rich in the class of fatty acids known as omega-6 fatty acids. These fatty acids create the inflammatory group of prostaglandins. Incidentally, aspirin and other NSAIDs block the formation of this group of prostaglandins. This is how they act to control pain and relieve inflammation.

FISH OILS

Q   **What kinds of fats are anti-inflammatory?**

A   Oils and fats are a class of substance known as triglycerides. Each molecule consists of a kind of backbone of glycerine (glycerol) to which are attached three fatty acids. During digestion the fatty acids are separated from the glycerol. Two kinds of oils seem to be anti-inflammatory: those containing **omega-3 fatty acids** (also called **eicosapentaenoic acid**, or **EPA**) found in fatty fish; and those containing **gamma-linolenic acid (GLA)**, found in high concentrations in blackcurrant oil, evening-primrose oil and borage oil.

Q I've heard a lot lately about fish oils. What are they?

A Oils containing omega-3 fatty acids are found mostly in cold-water fatty fish such as mackerel, sardines and salmon. They're also found in purslane, a fleshy weed that's easily grown in home vegetable gardens. Omega-3 fatty acids are liquid at room temperature and remain liquid even at very low temperatures.

You've probably heard about them in conjunction with heart disease. They have been found to reduce the clotting tendency in blood, and so to lower risk of heart attack. They've also been shown to inhibit inflammation by interfering with the production of inflammatory prostaglandins and altering certain aspects of the immune system.

Q How do they help people with rheumatoid arthritis?

A Six studies have been done so far to examine the effects of omega-3 fatty acids on people with rheumatoid arthritis. All have shown a modest beneficial effect. One of these studies compared people with active RA who took high or low doses of omega-3 fish oils with those who took olive oil. Both the high and low fish-oil groups saw more of an improvement in symptoms than the olive-oil group saw. But the high-dose fish-oil group did best, improving in 21 out of 45 clinical measures, including grip strength, number of swollen joints and the length of time they could remain active without becoming tired.

In these studies, the people who took fish oil also continued to take their arthritis medication. Improvement in symptoms is not usually seen until after at least 12 weeks of continuous use and appears to increase with extended treatment intervals of 18 to 24 weeks.

Doses have varied from study to study, and the research has not yet shown the ideal dosage and formulation, or even whether fish oils should be used to supplement or to replace certain parts of the traditional RA drug regimen.

Q **What about gamma-linolenic acid?**

A Gamma-linolenic acid, also liquid at room temperature, is found in concentrated amounts in blackcurrant oil, evening-primrose oil and borage oil. It, too, seems to inhibit inflammation by suppressing the production of biochemicals that cause inflammation. However, this oil has been studied less than have the omega-3 fatty acids.

In a study at the Royal Infirmary in Glasgow, doctors found that gamma-linolenic acid, alone or in combination with omega-3 fish oils, gave a number of people with mild rheumatoid arthritis enough pain relief to allow them to stop taking their nonsteroidal anti-inflammatory drugs.

One group of people in this study took 12 capsules a day of evening-primrose oil. Another group took a combination of fish oil and evening-primrose oil. A third group took a harmless look-alike capsule of paraffin.

At the end of three months, all the patients tried to cut down on their drugs, but were told to do so only if their symptoms did not worsen. Of the 28 patients who were able to stop or reduce their drugs, 11 were taking evening-primrose oil at the time, and 12 were taking the combination of fish oil and evening-primrose oil.

Q So what does all this mean to me in terms of my diet?

A Doctors who are incorporating these findings into their dietary recommendations for people with rheumatoid arthritis suggest the following:

- Make sure you eat enough to maintain your normal body weight. This is something many people with RA often fail to do, either because they're avoiding foods they think are causing symptoms, taking drugs that cause nausea or gastrointestinal upset, or have limited mobility which makes it hard for them to shop or cook.
- Make sure you are getting the Recommended Dietary Allowance (RDA) of every nutrient, which is hard to do even when you are active and are eating a high-calorie diet. You may want to take a multi-vitamin/mineral and individual supplements as necessary. The RDA is the amount of a nutrient deemed adequate for preventing nutritional deficiency-related diseases.
- Keep your total fat intake fairly low, getting about 25 per cent of calories from fat. This means you should eat plenty of grains and vegetables and stick with lean cuts of meat and low-fat dairy foods.
- Reduce your intake of safflower, sunflower, corn, sesame or soy oil by cutting back on salad dressings, fried foods and margarine.
- Increase your intake of fish oil. The safest, easiest way to do this is by eating three meals a week of

fatty fish. If you want to take fish-oil capsules, discuss dosage with your doctor.

Some doctors also recommend that you increase your intake of gamma-linolenic acid by taking capsules containing this oil. Gamma-linolenic acid does not occur in large amounts in any commonly eaten food, so it's hard to come by in most diets. Other doctors don't think there is enough research yet to validate making this recommendation.

Q **Do I need medical supervision to make these dietary modifications?**

A Some doctors say yes, others no. We recommend you consult your doctor before you make any major changes to your diet, including adding fish oils or gamma-linolenic acid. In studies so far, these oils seem to be safe. However, researchers point out that no one knows the possible risks associated with long-term, high-dose use of these oils.

VITAMINS AND MINERALS

Q **What about vitamins and minerals? Do any in particular help arthritis?**

A Here again, there's a lack of solid research. But to answer your question, so far no one vitamin or mineral seems to stand out as having a significant impact on on either rheumatoid arthritis or osteoarthritis.

Some vitamins and minerals, such as calcium,

selenium and vitamin C, are known to be involved in the formation of bone, cartilage and connective tissue, or in the formation of biochemicals which have anti-inflammatory properties in the body. There is also speculation that some play a role in rheumatoid arthritis, osteoarthritis or inflammation in general. These are all good reasons to make sure you are getting the RDA of every essential nutrient.

Q **I've heard it's important for people with arthritis to take plenty of vitamin C. Is this true?**

A It may well be. Inflammation tends to deplete the body's stores of vitamin C. Compounding the problem, nonsteroidal anti-inflammatory drugs interfere with vitamin C metabolism and excretion. Research also shows that people with rheumatoid arthritis have significantly lower blood levels of vitamin C than people without RA, irrespective of drug therapy. For these reasons, some doctors recommend higher-than-normal doses of vitamin C for their patients with RA – 3,000 milligrams (3 g) a day of vitamin C, 50 times the RDA, is by no means an unusual recommended dose for this vitamin. Research has shown that vitamin C is remarkably safe, even in large amounts. Do not be misled by this, however, into thinking that you can safely take 50 times the normal dose of other vitamins. Overdosage, especially of vitamins A and D, is very dangerous.

In one study, British researchers who gave 500 mg of vitamin C daily to people with rheumatoid arthritis found a dramatic lessening of the bruising frequently associated with RA. In another study, supplemental vitamin C perked up sluggish immune response in people with RA. Other studies, however, have found no effect on the course of rheumatoid arthritis, either with large daily doses or with injections of vitamin C directly into the joint.

Vitamins C and E are antioxidants and have been shown to be effective in dealing with the free radicals that are at the heart of so much tissue damage in a wide range of disease processes. It is still too early to say whether an attack on free radicals by adequate dosage of antioxidant vitamins will be useful in arthritis.

Q **Are people with arthritis low in any other nutrients?**
A Yes. Perhaps because they're so often malnourished, people with RA often have quite a few nutritional deficiencies.

A study by Finnish researchers showed reduced blood levels in people with RA for vitamins A and E, along with zinc. All three of these nutrients play a role in immune function and may help to control inflammation in the body.

In one study, large doses of zinc (50 mg, three times a day) improved symptoms in 12 out of 24 people with RA. These people had not responded well to other forms of treatment. In another study, zinc supplementation improved some symptoms in people with psoriatic arthritis (inflammatory arthritis coupled with the skin disease psoriasis). However, another study showed no improvement after zinc supplementation in people with long-standing RA.

Q Do doctors make any recommendations about these nutrients?

A Here again, some researchers suggest that rheumatoid arthritis sufferers eat foods rich in vitamin E, zinc and beta-carotene (a plant substance converted to vitamin A in the body). Others, concerned with the use of vitamins as antioxidants, recommend daily intakes of 1,500 to 3,000 mg of vitamin C, 30 mg of beta-carotene, and 400 IU of vitamin E.

Q Are there other nutrients which people with RA are low in?

A Yes. A study found that blood levels of pantothenic acid, a B-complex vitamin, were significantly lower in people with RA than in healthy people. Studies with animals have shown that young rats acutely deficient in pantothenic acid suffer defects in growth and development of bone and cartilage. Two British studies have looked at supplementation of pantothenic acid in people with RA. In both studies, supplementation led to some improvement in symptoms. This finding should be viewed with some scepticism, however; there is no evidence that pantothenic acid deficiency ever occurs in humans.

Selenium, a trace mineral involved in immune-system functioning – and which may act both as an anti-inflammatory and a pro-inflammatory – has also been found to be low in people with RA. Injected and oral selenium and vitamin E preparations are used in veterinary practice to relieve arthritic inflammation in dogs and other animals. Results are reported to be good. Unfortunately, there are no good studies of its use in people with RA. The body's requirement for selenium is very small indeed, and it is extremely rare, almost unheard of, for deficiency to occur. A daily 50 mcg supplement (a microgram is one-millionth of a gram) of selenium has been recommended to people with RA. Note, however, that more is definitely not better when it comes to selenium. Large amounts are toxic.

Vitamin B_6 supplements are sometimes recommended to people with RA, especially if they suffer from carpal tunnel syndrome, a pinched nerve in the wrist, or tarsal tunnel syndrome, the same problem in the ankle. In several small studies, vitamin B_6 reduced pain and symptoms of numbness in some people with carpal or tarsal tunnel syndrome. Large doses of vitamin B_6 can cause nerve problems, however, and this vitamin should be taken only under medical supervision.

Studies also indicate that people with RA have depressed iron levels and mild anaemia, due in part to problems the body has using its stores of iron – probably because of disease. Usually this anaemia does not respond to iron therapy. Intravenous infusions of an iron-sugar solution in RA patients were observed to precipitate flare-ups, which has led some researchers to raise the possibility that excessive quantities of iron may be harmful in people with inflammatory diseases.

So the use of iron supplementation in people with RA is controversial. Some doctors believe it should be avoided.

Q **What about copper – and copper bracelets?**

A The official word from the medical establishment on copper bracelets is 'just plain silly'. One major survey of patients who tried some sort of copper jewellery – 211 out of 1,051 – didn't find it particularly helpful. Some 85 per cent said it did nothing, 6 per cent said it helped, and another 7 per cent said it may have helped. This is the sort of result to be expected from a 'remedy' that actually has no effect.

One Australian study looked at copper bracelets and arthritis. In this study, 240 'arthritis/rheumatism' sufferers were randomly assigned to one of three groups. Group I wore a copper bracelet for one month followed by a placebo bracelet (aluminium) for one month. Group II wore the two bracelets in reverse order, while Group III wore no bracelets at all. Of the 77 people who completed the study, 47 claimed that they noticed a difference between the bracelets. Some 37 of these 47 believed that the copper one was more effective. These researchers also found that copper bracelets decrease in weight after they're worn for a while, which could mean that copper is being absorbed from the bracelet into the body. The real trouble with this study was that since copper bracelets are widely believed to have therapeutic value, one would expect participants to attribute subjective improvement to the bracelets.

So the bottom line is this: wear one if you want, but don't count on it to relieve your symptoms. And certainly don't count on it to cure your arthritis. Above all, don't abandon other treatments that do work.

Q   **What about copper in my diet? Is it important?**

A   Copper is thought to play a role in rheumatoid arthritis. Just what role this might be isn't understood. Researchers know that copper levels are elevated in both the blood and synovial fluid of people with RA, but they don't know if that means the body is mobilizing copper stores to fight inflammation.

Q   **What else is known?**

A   The plain truth is that a great deal of nonsense is talked and written about the role of copper in disease. Copper is a very minor player in the biochemical league. At present there is really no basis for the large claims made for copper in that segment of the popular medical press in which critical standards have been displaced by enthusiasm.

Q   **I'm still worried that I might not be getting enough copper. What are good food sources of copper?**

A   Liver, oysters, crab meat, sesame and sunflower seeds, and nuts all contain good amounts of copper. Remember, though, as with other trace minerals, large doses of copper are toxic. You should take copper supplements only under medical supervision.

Q   **You said earlier that taking NSAIDs can increase a person's need for vitamin C. Do any other arthritis drugs deplete your body of particular nutrients?**

A   Methotrexate, a drug used for RA, actually works by depleting the body of a B-complex vitamin, folic acid. Some studies show that adding folic acid reduces methotrexate's side-effects without affecting the drug's effectiveness.

People with RA taking nonsteroidal anti-inflammatory drugs have been found to have reduced blood levels of zinc.

Steroid drugs, too, such as prednisolone, tend to deplete bone mass, especially if they are taken in large doses or over a long period of time. To attempt to counteract this, some doctors tell their patients on steroids to get extra amounts of calcium and vitamin D.

Finally, penicillamine, gold and steroids may all interfere with the body's ability to absorb and use selenium and other trace minerals, including copper.

Q   **So far you've talked only about rheumatoid arthritis. What are the dietary recommendations for people with osteoarthritis?**

A   The top dietary recommendation for osteoarthritis is to maintain your normal weight. Several population studies have shown a link between obesity and the development of osteoarthritis, mostly in the weight-bearing joints, the hips and knees, and even the feet and ankles.

Q **What exactly is this link?**

A If you are too heavy these joints are going to be exposed to considerable pressure. Standing on one leg applies about three times the total body weight on the hip, knee and ankle joints. Walking up or down stairs puts roughly six times the body weight on these joints. So every extra pound counts.

A knee joint can actually be compressed as a result of extra weight, making the cartilage-lined bones grind against each other and causing excessive wear and tear. Heavy thighs can contribute to pain by forcing you to stand with your feet far apart and your toes pointed out. That stance throws your joints out of alignment and adds stress to hips and knees.

Q **Can losing weight prevent osteoarthritis?**

A A recent study indicates that it can. Researchers reviewed the weight histories of 64 women recently diagnosed with osteoarthritis of the knee, and 728 women without the condition. All the women had been weighed frequently as participants in the ongoing Framingham Study, that has followed the health of the residents of Framingham, Massachusetts, for 44 years. The study showed that an overweight woman of average height (5 ft 3 in) who loses 11 pounds over a 10-year-period can reduce her risk of developing knee arthritis by more than half. And women who lose more weight decrease their arthritis risk even further.

Clearly many overweight women could delay or even prevent osteoarthritis of the knees by losing weight.

Q **But can losing weight help people who already have osteoarthritis?**

A There are no good studies to prove that losing weight lessens joint pain or slows the progress of the disease in people who already have osteoarthritis. But the experience of doctors who treat people with osteoarthritis is that weight loss does help, simply by taking the squeeze off overburdened joints. This isn't going to work, however, unless the person concerned is at least 20 per cent above ideal weight and the weight loss is substantial. It is estimated that you have to lose at least half your excess weight to derive any useful effect. Don't let that discourage you, however. Losing excess weight has so many medical advantages that nothing should be allowed to stand in your way of achieving it.

Q **I've heard that people who are severely overweight often don't do well with artificial joints. Is this true?**

A In general they don't seem to do as well as people of normal weight. Surgeons have been reluctant to do joint replacements in people who are very heavy, because cemented joints are more likely to loosen in overweight people. The rate of complications after joint replacement rises steeply in people weighing more than 13 stone (180 lb). It may be that the new cementless joints will prove to be less of a problem in overweight people, but so far there hasn't been enough time to prove this.

Q   **What about people with rheumatoid arthritis? Does losing weight ever help them?**

A   As we said earlier, people with RA tend to be underweight. Studies show that those who are overweight, however, do seem to increase their risk of joint damage. So it's probable that they, too, would benefit from weight loss.

Q   **You've talked so much about fish oils and rheumatoid arthritis – do fish oils provide any benefit for people with osteoarthritis?**

A   Osteoarthritis is much less likely than rheumatoid arthritis to be associated with inflammation, and that's why fish oils and evening-primrose oil aren't usually recommended for this condition. But in one small study, British researchers did try adding fish oil to some of their osteoarthritic patients' regular treatments with ibuprofen. At four months, the people taking the fish oil reported a 'strikingly lower' assessment of pain and interference with daily activities than the patients taking ibuprofen alone.

Q   **What about the nutrients you mentioned earlier that help keep bones strong or are important for cartilage formation? Can they do anything for osteoarthritis?**

A   Here again, evidence is scant, and many of the studies that have been done over the years simply aren't up to the rigorous standards today's medical community demands as proof that something works. Rather than looking for one particular nutrient to cure your disease, your best bet is to make sure you really are getting an adequately balanced diet. Many nutrients are important for bone health: calcium, vitamins D, C and B_6, as well as traces of many minerals.

Vitamin C has proven helpful, in an animal study, in preventing cartilage damage. And vitamin C has been found to increase cartilage cell growth in rabbits. Vitamin E was found helpful in relieving pain from osteoarthritis in a study by Israeli researchers. More than half of the 32 patients taking 600 IU of vitamin E a day for 10 days experienced marked relief of pain, according to this study. The antioxidant role of these two vitamins has been attracting increasing medical attention in connection with a wide range of diseases other than arthritis.

Q   **Aren't there nutritional supplements I can take to help my body rebuild cartilage?**

A   There are substances being sold with the claim that they can rebuild cartilage, but again, sadly, the proof that they work is not such as would satisfy critical scientists. Substances such as green-lipped mussels, shark cartilage and calf cartilage, along with a substance called **chondroitin sulphate**, all contain building blocks for cartilage – **glycosaminoglycans**. Chondroitin sulphate is available in some health-food shops. Some studies claim to have shown benefits in restoring damaged cartilage, both with oral and injected forms of chondroitin sulphate. The jury is still out, however, on this one.

OTHER ALTERNATIVE TREATMENTS

Q **Isn't there some sort of liquid that people put on their joints to ease the pain?**

A You're talking about DMSO, which is short for dimethyl sulphoxide. DMSO has been used since the 1940s as an industrial solvent, and was introduced into therapeutic practice in the 1960s. It was studied by researchers for a time for a variety of problems, ranging from athletic injuries to rheumatoid arthritis.

DMSO is odourless and colourless, but once applied to a joint it can leave your breath smelling of garlic, onions or worse. Many claims have been made as to its proposed modes of action, but none of these claims has been widely accepted.

One survey found that DMSO provided temporary relief of joint pain in about half of the 47 people who tried it. It is not recommended, though, since it does not outperform standard arthritis treatments, and it has not been proven to affect the course of the disease. Don't be tempted to buy commercial-grade DMSO and try it yourself. If you do want to use it, discuss the matter first with your doctor, who may agree to prescribe medical-grade DMSO.

After a review of the research studies done on DMSO, a special committee of the American National Academy of Sciences found DMSO too 'iffy' and risky to become a prescription drug, much less an over-the-counter drug. In animals, DMSO has caused damage to the lens of the eye. Moreover, there are still no studies to prove that DMSO does anything worthwhile to help arthritis.

Q **What about bee venom? I've heard some people with rheumatoid arthritis are treated with it.**

A Bee venom has a long history of use as a folk remedy for inflammatory conditions such as rheumatoid arthritis. But there are no controlled clinical studies proving it works. There are some anecdotal reports and uncontrolled studies, however, that indicate benefits.

One author points out, rather paradoxically, that bee venom is rich in anti-inflammatory substances. Tell that to someone who has just been stung by a bee! Some minor trials have been done, with inconclusive results. You are unlikely to be able to find an orthodox doctor willing to treat you in this way, but there are alternative practitioners who will provide you with a series of injections over the course of months, in slowly increasing amounts. After about six visits you may be receiving as many as 20 to 30 injections per visit. Alternatively, of course, you could take up beekeeping.

Q   **What about acupuncture? A friend of mine gets acupuncture treatments once a week and says they have eased her osteoarthritis pain.**

A   Acupuncture is a traditional Chinese therapy that involves inserting very fine, sterilized needles into certain areas of the body. It's not considered painful and the risks are mainly those of infection if the needles are not properly sterilized. Some practitioners use disposable needles. There is also a slight risk that a needle will break off in the tissues. Such needles can be very difficult to retrieve.

Acupuncture does seem to have pain-relieving effects, although just how it works isn't fully understood. Some researchers believe it stimulates the body's production of natural painkillers or anti-inflammatory biochemicals. Other say it closes physiological 'pain gates' through which pain nerve impulses are passing up to the brain. Acupuncturists say it stimulates the flow of 'vital energy' along certain energy meridians in the body to restore energy imbalances by 'unblocking' these meridians.

Q   **Is there any proof that acupuncture works?**

A   A recent study by Danish researchers compared the pain-relieving abilities of acupuncture with standard drug therapy in a group of 29 people with severe knee osteoarthritis who were candidates for knee replacement surgery. Half the patients were randomly assigned to receive acupuncture treatment; the other half received standard painkillers.

The researchers measured pain relief and knee function, including the time it took to walk 50 feet and climb 20 steps on a staircase. They also measured range of motion and muscle strength. After nine weeks, the people receiving acupuncture treatments had significantly less pain and better function than those on analgesics, according to the researchers. In fact, seven people responded so well they declined surgery. These researchers followed 17 of the initial 29 patients, continuing to give them acupuncture once a month for a year. With some ups and down, these patients were able to maintain the improvements seen at the beginning of the treatment.

While this all sounds good, critics say these results need to be repeated in other studies before this treatment can be considered proven to work. One of the problems is that the meridians have no physical existence. The whole scheme of energy flow along meridians is theoretical. It may be a metaphor, but it is not one that can be fitted into the scientific facts of anatomy and physiology.

Q How do I find someone who does acupuncture treatments?

A Unfortunately, anyone can set up as an acupuncturist regardless of medical knowledge or training, so be careful. Consult the Council for Acupuncture, 179 Gloucester Place, London NW1 6VX, tel. 0171–724 5756. They will provide you with a copy of the Directory of British Acupuncturists, all of whom have had accredited training and apply strict rules of ethics and practice.

Q **Do any herbal remedies help arthritis?**
A No doubt many have been tried, but here again there are few controlled clinical trials to prove that they work.

One remedy that has caught researchers' attention is a Chinese herb called *Triptergium wilfordii*, or thundervine root. In a study by researchers at Peking Union Medical College Hospital, in Beijing, this herb showed encouraging activity in people with rheumatoid arthritis. An extract of the plant achieved a 90 per cent reduction in pain and other RA symptoms in 30 patients who were treated for 12 weeks. A control group receiving harmless placebos showed only 23 per cent improvement. The observable clinical benefits were accompanied by improvements in the biochemical factors associated with RA, including rheumatoid factor and some measures of immune function.

There were some side-effects, however, from the thundervine extract – mainly skin rashes and mild diarrhoea. Several of the women found that the drug stopped their menstrual periods. In a few postmenopausal women, the drug brought on bleeding. Chinese researchers will continue to look at this herb, hoping to isolate its helpful components.

Q **Can herbs be dangerous?**
A They certainly can. Just like drugs, all herbs, essential oils and extracts can contain active ingredients that cause

serious side-effects if not used properly. There has been at least one confirmed case where a remedy being marketed as 'Chinese herbs' turned out to include more than just herbs – when analysed, the 'remedy' was found to contain indomethacin, a strong anti-inflammatory drug with a long list of potential side-effects, and prednisone, a steroid drug with its own possible side-effects.

Also worrying is the total lack of standardization of many herbal remedies. Official drugs are carefully purified and standardized so that dispensed medication contains an exact amount of a particular substance. This is far from the case with herbal remedies. Variations from plant to plant, the effects of different seasonal growths and so on can result in any one preparation containing hundreds of times more or less than the intended dose. In these circumstances a prescribed or recommended dose can be meaningless. There is growing literature in the medical press about the harm that has been done to patients by herbal remedies, and there are increasing calls for its regularization in the UK.

EXPERIMENTAL TREATMENTS

Q **What's considered an experimental treatment? How does it differ from an alternative treatment such as acupuncture?**

A Most researchers consider an experimental treatment one that is being actively investigated in controlled clinical trials. A controlled trial is a study in which one group of people get the treatment being studied, while a similar group, the control group, gets either a placebo treatment or the standard treatment. Researchers consider an alternative treatment one that has not been investigated in any proper, organized manner in accordance with scientific protocol.

The borderline between the two may sometimes be narrow. In a few cases, a treatment which for a long time has been considered alternative, such as megavitamin C therapy or fish oils, may move into the experimental category and eventually be shown to be useful.

Q **What kinds of experimental treatments are being investigated now for arthritis?**

A There are many different areas of study. They include the development of what are called **biological agents** – medicinal preparations derived from living organisms which are administered in the same manner as drugs and which alter the body's immune response; new drugs that fight inflammation, hopefully with fewer side-effects than the drugs currently being used; drugs already approved for use which may also be effective against arthritis; and even biochemical agents which may stimulate cartilage regrowth.

Arthritis research has benefited greatly from basic immunological research directed towards the management of cancer and organ transplantation. Some anticancer drugs and those used to prevent the rejection of organ transplants are being tried in people with rheumatoid arthritis. As we have seen, methotrexate was first used as a cancer drug before it was tried, in much smaller doses, as a treatment for rheumatoid arthritis. **Cyclosporine**, a drug used extensively to prevent rejection in organ-transplant patients, has been used with some success in people with rheumatoid arthritis who haven't responded well to other treatments.

Q Sounds as though there are many research studies going on. Is this the case?

A Nobody knows exactly how many studies of experimental treatments for arthritis are being conducted at any one time. One reason for this is that drug and biotechnology companies – those producing the biological agents – tend to be secretive about what they're studying. They don't want their competitors stealing their ideas.

Q How does someone become involved in a research study?

A The best way to find out about research projects is to ask your rheumatologist. Although quite a number of GPs are involved in drug trial research, most research is conducted by hospital specialists. The chances are that your rheumatologist will either be involved in a research study or will know of some ongoing research in which you might become involved. Don't forget, however, that this may involve you in more attendances in hospital than would otherwise be necessary.

Q **How can I evaluate an experimental treatment?**

A By law, the researchers are required to discuss in detail the possible risks involved in any research study, and their study in particular, with anyone considering enroling in a study.

Because the research study will focus on an experimental treatment, there may not be much published about it. Still, you'll want to know what has been published, including animal studies and studies by foreign researchers. You should ask how long the new treatment has been studied, how many studies have been done, where it has been studied (at any teaching hospitals or universities?), how many people have used the treatment to date, if you were the first, what any previous studies have found in terms of benefits, what kinds of side-effects are possible, whether there have been any deaths associated with the treatment and how much precisely the researchers know (and don't yet know) about it.

Remember also that new is not necessarily better. Although some promising treatments seem to be in the pipeline, experience has proved that there are always a few that don't work out. As one researcher puts it, 'A lot of treatments look promising at the start, but many are found to have problems that limit their use.' Clinical trials are designed to uncover at least some of these problems.

Many researchers think biological agents hold the most hope for specific and effective therapies for rheumatoid arthritis, perhaps even a cure. So let's look at them first.

Q What exactly is a biological agent?

A It is a medicinal preparation (researchers call them agents, not drugs) made from living organisms and their products. Most are derived from mouse or human immune cells.

All the biological agents being studied for arthritis are intended to have some sort of effect on the body's immune system: either to restore normal function, to alter function or to suppress a function.

Q What are biological agents supposed to do in the case of RA?

A Unfortunately, no one knows for sure what biological agents need to do in order to be effective against RA and other rheumatic diseases, so researchers are trying all sorts of biologicals with all sorts of immune-system actions. Most biological agents, however, have some sort of effect on T-cells (immune cells that play an important role in the inflammatory process of RA).

One reason for the confusion is that no one knows exactly how the immune system works in the case of RA, so no one knows for sure which immune-system functions need to be altered to have an impact on this disease. As always in medical research, what is needed is a clear understanding of the nature and causation of the underlying disease processes (the pathology). Once the pathology is fully known, a logical attack nearly always becomes possible, often very quickly.

Q   **What sorts of biological agents are being tried right now?**

A   One that's gone through at least eight clinical trials with RA patients is **gamma-interferon**, a biological agent that's used in another form (alpha) as a treatment for some types of cancer.

Gamma-interferon is a protein produced by certain of the body's immune cells when they are invaded by viruses. Interferon itself is not an antiviral agent, but it acts to stimulate uninfected cells, causing them to make another protein with antiviral characteristics. Interferons and other substances that act in a similar way (called interleukins) can also be produced by cells in response to a wide variety of stimulants, including bacterial invasion or bacterial toxin. Interferons and interleukins have a wide range of effects on the body's immune system. Unfortunately, their role in rheumatoid arthritis remains unclear.

In studies in which gamma-interferon has been given to people with rheumatoid arthritis, results have been mixed. In these studies, improvement in symptoms of joint swelling and pain ranged from 15 to 60 per cent.

Q   **Is there any other new research?**

A   Another area of research is in **monoclonal antibodies**. An antibody, you'll recall, is a type of blood protein made by the body in response to a foreign substance (called an antigen). An antibody binds to an antigen and eliminates it from the body. Monoclonal antibodies, selected for a particular purpose, can be produced in a lab in large quantities by persuading particular B cells (the cells that produce antibodies) to form tumours.

Arthritis researchers are interested in certain types of monoclonal antibodies because they seem to be capable of blocking inflammatory reactions by certain cells, including cells in the joint capsule. Unlike most anti-inflammatory drugs used for arthritis, monoclonal antibodies seem to provide their beneficial effects right at the source of the action – certain immune cells which get into a joint and produce inflammation.

Just how well monoclonal antibody therapy may work for RA has yet to be determined. Studies done so far, with a variety of antibodies, have been encouraging.

Q   **What other kinds of biological agents are being tried?**
A   There are several, but one type in particular – **immuno-toxins** – have caught researchers' interest. Immuno-toxins start out as monoclonal antibodies but are combined with a poison so that when they attach to a cell's surface they destroy the cell. So far, immunotoxins have been designed to destroy certain kinds of T-cells, which, as we said earlier, are immune cells that play a major role in inflammation. It may be possible, however, to design an immunotoxin which can destroy any type of cell.

In one Harvard University study, 12 of 13 people with severe rheumatoid arthritis who had not responded to other therapies showed a significant response to an immunotoxin containing deactivated diphtheria toxin. Studies of immunotoxins are ongoing, but researchers say it's too soon to know if these agents can provide long-term relief.

Q **What about anti-inflammatory drugs? Are there any safer, more effective ones being developed?**

A We don't know about safer or more effective, but there certainly are a lot of anti-inflammatory drugs being marketed, and manufacturers keep coming out with more.

A considerable number of new anti-inflammatory drugs are currently being tested or are awaiting official approval to be marketed. To be given approval, a drug must prove that it is at least as safe and effective as those in the same category already on the market. So clinical trials must compare the drug with others in its class.

One potentially important new anti-inflammatory drug, tenidap, has aroused a great deal of interest. Currently it is licensed in the Netherlands and Spain, but is still awaiting approval in the UK. This drug seems to be the start of a new class of anti-inflammatory medications. Its chemical structure is unlike that of any existing drugs used to treat RA. It seems to be unique among anti-rheumatics in that it has a dual anti-inflammatory action. In addition to inhibiting the body's manufacture of inflammatory prostaglandins, the drug acts on immune cells called neutrophils which, when activated, release biochemicals that can damage cells. Neutrophils are the predominant cells in synovial fluid, and are frequently found in areas where inflamed, proliferating synovial tissue is pressing against cartilage.

This drug has more than held its own against other popular NSAIDs, and is currently being extensively tested in a large trial of 10,000 people. Over 2,000 patients with rheumatoid arthritis have already received tenidap, and these trials suggest that its effectiveness is equivalent to that of gold or hydroxychloroquine plus an NSAID. Adverse reactions were found to be similar to those caused by NSAIDs alone. Further study should show whether or not this drug helps to alter the progressive joint damage so commonly seen in patients with arthritis. Tenidap is currently being considered for use in both osteoarthritis and rheumatoid arthritis.

Q I've read something about tetracycline being tried in people with rheumatoid arthritis. What's the story behind this?

A Researchers are now testing a form of the antibiotic tetracycline, called **minocycline**, on 219 people with rheumatoid arthritis.

An Israeli study tested minocycline in people with rheumatoid arthritis and found significant improvements in almost all aspects of the disease.

Antibiotics have been tried, off and on, for the treatment of arthritis for about 30 years, but so far studies of their effectiveness have been mixed. It now appears that these drugs, if effective, are not working as antibiotics but as modulators of the immune system. It is thought that minocycline reduces inflammation by inhibiting an enzyme involved in dissolving cartilage in the joint. Minocycline may prove to be useful for the treatment of

RA, but, like other drugs, it does have side-effects. Dizziness, nausea and rashes were most commonly reported by the Israeli researchers. And, of course, there is always the risk with long-term use of antibiotics that antibiotic-resistant germs may develop in the body. In the Israeli study, three people developed either oral or skin candida (thrush) infections.

CHAPTER FIVE

OTHER QUESTIONS ABOUT ARTHRITIS

Q   **What exactly is rheumatism?**

A   It's an imprecise term people use to describe just about any condition which causes pain and swelling in joints and surrounding tissues. Rheumatism may be diagnosed as arthritis, bursitis or any other of a number of painful conditions.

Q   **My friend claims her rheumatoid arthritis has improved since she started oestrogen-replacement therapy. Is there any proof this should help?**

A   One American study by researchers at the University of California at San Francisco found that women with rheumatoid arthritis who take oestrogen-replacement therapy have milder symptoms than women who took oestrogen in the past but stopped or who never used oestrogen.

The study, of 154 postmenopausal women with RA, found that use of hormone replacement therapy was associated with significantly fewer painful joints and better performance of daily activities.

Sex hormones are steroids, known to influence immune response and the course of autoimmune diseases. Such diseases are more common in women of reproductive age. Just what role sex hormones may play in rheumatoid arthritis remains to be determined, researchers say. Pregnancy improves RA symptoms. And some evidence suggests that the use of oral contraceptives can reduce a woman's lifetime risk of RA, or at least delay its onset.

Q **But aren't there risks associated with hormone replacement therapy?**

A Yes, so you'll need to be monitored by your doctor if you decide to take oestrogen and other replacement hormones.

Oestrogen, when taken alone in any form, increases a woman's risk of developing cancer of the endometrium – the uterine lining. So a woman should take an additional hormone, progesterone, which causes the uterine lining to be shed each month. If she does not take progesterone, her doctor should occasionally take a sample of endometrium to make sure it is normal.

Studies that look at the risk of breast cancer in women taking hormone replacement hormones have been mixed. Most have found no increased risk. One study, however, found a slightly increased risk of 10 per cent overall, and also found several high-risk groups. Women who took a combination of oestrogen and progesterone for more than six years, for instance, appeared to have about four times the average risk of developing breast cancer. That was a very small group, though, and doctors say additional research is needed to learn more about the risks of such long-term therapy. A doctor will probably recommend a yearly mammogram for any woman undergoing hormone replacement therapy.

Q   **Will moving to a warmer climate help my arthritis?**
A   Studies on the effect of weather on rheumatoid arthritis show that when barometric pressure goes down and humidity goes up, the symptoms of arthritis worsen for some people. And many people say their joints feel better when the weather is warm and dry than when it's cold and damp.

   The weather itself doesn't cause arthritis, however, and it's unlikely that moving to a warmer, drier climate will alter the course of the disease, although it may make you feel more comfortable. Before you decide to move, it's a good idea to visit the place you have in mind for a few weeks to see if you really do feel better being there. Some people with arthritis who move to a new climate find that the disadvantages of giving up their ties to family and friends outweigh the advantages of a sunny clime.

Q   **Is there a connection between stress and arthritis?**
A   There does seem to be a connection, researchers are discovering. How secure this is scientifically is another matter. It is very common for people with rheumatoid arthritis to relate the onset of their symptoms to a particularly stressful period in their lives, or to say their symptoms flare up when they are feeling stressed. This,

however, is far from proving that the RA is caused by stress. Increasingly, links between stress and the functioning of the immune system are being discovered.

Q **How might stress play a role in arthritis?**

A One theory is that people who develop chronic inflammation may produce lower levels of corticosteroids. These are normally released by the adrenal glands in response to physical or emotional stress, and are the most powerful anti-inflammatory agents produced by the body. If a person is unable to produce normal amounts of corticosteroids, it seems probable that inflammatory diseases may develop.

Q **How can I find out if I have a stress-hormone deficiency myself?**

A It is possible to have a test that measures your blood levels of stress hormones, but it is by no means certain that the test results would enable your doctor to predict the course of your RA or usefully modify your treatment. Testing standards which would associate certain blood levels of stress hormones with symptoms of inflammation have yet to be developed.

Q **So what can I do if I think stress is contributing to my symptoms?**

A Researchers say this:

- Don't be embarrassed to mention to your doctor that your condition varies with the amount of stress you feel.

- Avoid what stressful situations you can. Stress counselling or biofeedback may help you react less to stressful situations.
- Based on the theory that many people with RA may have a stress-hormone deficiency, some doctors prescribe what they call physiological doses (3 to 4 mg a day) of steroid drugs. They allow their patients to assess their own degree of inflammation and determine their own dosage. There is little doubt that such doses work fairly well at relieving symptoms, but many doctors disapprove of using steroids in this way.
- Some doctors also prescribe antidepressants, which often seem to help. They may even normalize either overproduction or underproduction of natural corticosteroids.

Q   **Does depression have something to do with RA?**

A   Researchers say it's common for people with rheumatoid arthritis to have what's called *atypical depression*, a form characterized by foul moods, lack of energy and excessive sleep. This is not particularly surprising. RA is a serious, painful and disabling disease, and depression is quite a normal reaction. There is some evidence, however, that this depression may be caused by the same stress-hormone deficiency that increases people's susceptibility to inflammatory illnesses. Some doctors are currently studying which types of antidepressants are most likely to help people with atypical depression.

Q **Can I have osteoarthritis and rheumatoid arthritis at the same time?**

A Yes. Joints damaged by rheumatoid arthritis are prone to develop osteoarthritis, as are any injured joints. And RA-damaged weight-bearing joints, such as knees, are likely to develop osteoarthritis at an earlier than normal age. Both conditions need to be treated, using combinations of drugs that minimize RA flare-ups and relieve osteoarthritis pain, along with rest and non-weight-bearing exercises.

Q **You mentioned Lyme disease earlier. Tell me again – what exactly is it? What causes it?**

A Lyme disease is an infectious condition that can cause a number of medical problems, including arthritis, usually only in a few large joints.

It's caused by a spiral-shaped bacteria called *Borrelia burgdorferi* which is transmitted to humans by the bite of an animal tick, a tiny insect that in its immature state can fit on the head of a pin. Most people are bitten by immature ticks during spring and summer. Adult ticks are a little bigger and can bite at other times of the year. Deer are commonly infested with these ticks, but other animals also carry them.

Q **What are the symptoms of Lyme disease?**

A Its early symptoms can include a flu-like illness, with chills, fever, headache, swollen glands and joint pain. About half of infected people also develop a distinctive rash around the site of the tick bite within three days to a month after being bitten. The rash features a red ring with a clear centre. The outer edges expand slowly in size. Sometimes the centre of the ring becomes a large red blister. In many cases, multiple rings appear as a characteristic of the disease. These multiple rings are not at the sites of other tick bites.

If it is not treated, Lyme disease can cause severe nerve or heart problems, as well as arthritis.

Q   **How is Lyme disease diagnosed?**

A   Hopefully, your medical history and the appearance of the rash can provide your doctor with enough clues to be fairly certain of a diagnosis. However, if you don't recall being bitten by a tick and do not develop the classic red ring rash, diagnosis may be something of a challenge.

A number of blood tests can be done to test for Lyme disease. Most common are the indirect fluorescent antibody (IFA) test, the Western blot assay and the ELISA (enzyme-linked immunosorbent assay). All three measure antibodies in the blood formed against the bacteria that cause Lyme disease. However, studies have shown that all three of these tests are inaccurate in detecting Lyme disease 20 to 60 per cent of the time. Their false-positive or false-negative rates vary widely, depending in part on the laboratory at which they are done. That means you can't rely on a negative blood test to rule out the possibility that you have Lyme disease.

Q **Sounds like Lyme disease is often misdiagnosed. Is it?**

A It seems to be. Lyme disease is still fairly rare in Britain and Europe. It was first described in Lyme, Connecticut, and seems to be increasingly common in the US. Now increasing numbers of cases are being described on this side of the Atlantic. If you think you may have this disease, and especially if you are likely to have been in contact with animal ticks, you should be investigated in a teaching hospital.

Q **How is Lyme disease treated?**

A In the early stages of the disease, oral antibiotics, such as doxycycline, amoxicillin and erythromycin, are given for three to four weeks and are usually effective at curing the disease. Intravenous antibiotics are often necessary in its later stages, and some people develop chronic symptoms which some doctors treat with long-term intravenous antibiotics.

Q **What can I do to protect myself from being bitten?**

A Experts suggest that when outdoors you should wear tightly woven light-coloured clothing and tuck long trousers into socks. Lightly spray your clothing and skin, and especially your shoes, socks and lower legs with an insect repellent containing deet.

When you come indoors, or once each day if you're outside for days at a time, check your body, including your groin and underarms, for ticks. Ask someone to check your head and neck. Check your pets daily for ticks. If you do find a tick, grasp it with fine-point tweezers as close to the skin as possible and pull it straight out. Do not attempt to crush it with your fingers, as this may drive the hard shell into your skin. If possible, save the tick in a container filled with alcohol. That way, if you become ill, a doctor can identify the tick and more readily treat your illness.

If you know for sure you were bitten by a deer tick, some doctors suggest a preventive course of antibiotics even if you haven't developed symptoms.

Q   **What is fibromyalgia?**

A   This disorder literally means pain ('algia') in fibrous tissues, such as muscles, tendons and ligaments. It's also sometimes called fibrositis, but that name is misleading, since this condition does not involve inflammation. Some of its symptoms – chronic, diffuse aches and pains, disturbed sleep, morning fatigue and stiffness, headaches, numbness and/or tingling – are similar to those of arthritis, but standard arthritis treatments, such as nonsteroidal anti-inflammatory drugs, don't seem to help. Some 70 to 90 per cent of people who develop fibromyalgia are women aged 20 to 50.

Q   **How is fibromyalgia diagnosed?**

A   The diagnosis is made on the basis of physical symptoms and the elimination of other possible disorders, such as Lyme disease and rheumatoid arthritis.

People with fibromyalgia have what doctors call 'tender points' at specific locations throughout their bodies. These muscular nodules may not hurt normally, but pressing on them causes pain. Doctors look for multiple tender points, which are uncommon in healthy people and in people with other rheumatic diseases.

There is no blood test or laboratory test to identify the presence of fibromyalgia. X-rays reveal nothing.

Q **Do doctors know what causes it?**

A No, but there are several theories. Some researchers think the problem stems from sleep disturbances which lead to fatigue, pain and depression. Some think it's a problem of muscle energy metabolism, and that muscle cells starved for oxygen are causing the pain. Others think it is caused by various infections, thyroid disease, head trauma or emotional stress. In one study, half of the people with fibromyalgia said their symptoms began after a flu-like illness. Many had been diagnosed as having chronic-fatigue syndrome (ME). To confuse matters even more, some researchers think fibromyalgia and chronic-fatigue syndrome are the same condition.

Q **How is fibromyalgia treated?**

A Generally, non-drug treatments, such as heat, massage and muscle stretching, are tried first. Such treatments may be all some people require to relieve their symptoms. In one study, aerobic exercise was also helpful at relieving pain and improving sleep.

Antidepressants are the drugs used most often to treat fibromyalgia. This does not mean that people with fibromyalgia are depressed or have a psychiatric disorder. They are usually not depressed. Doctors prescribe these drugs, to be taken at bedtime, because they improve sleep and so eliminate some of the problems that poor sleep patterns can cause. In several studies, people taking antidepressants showed a significant improvement in symptoms.

Doctors say that narcotics and steroid drugs should never be given to people with fibromyalgia.

Q **You've mentioned lupus a few times. What can you tell me about this disease?**

A Like rheumatoid arthritis, lupus is a chronic inflammatory disease in which the body's immune system forms antibodies which attack healthy tissues and organs. There are several types of lupus. **Discoid lupus** affects the skin, causing a butterfly-shaped rash across the face and a rash on the upper parts of the body. Systemic lupus erythematosus (SLE), usually more severe than discoid, can attack any body part, such as the joints, kidneys, brain, heart or lungs. Like rheumatoid arthritis, lupus includes flare-ups and remissions. If not controlled, SLE can be dangerous. Another form of this disease is drug-induced lupus, caused by reactions to medication. When the drug is stopped, the symptoms of lupus usually disappear. It's not known how many people have discoid lupus. Probably many people have mild cases and don't know it.

Q   **What causes lupus?**

A   Only in the case of drug-induced lupus is the cause known. The drug most likely to be implicated is procainamide (Pronestyl), which is often used to treat heart irregularities. Other drugs known to cause lupus include hydralazine (a blood-pressure drug), isoniazid (used to treat tuberculosis), methyldopa (a blood-pressure drug), quinidine (used to treat heart irregularities) and chlorpromazine (used to treat psychosis and severe vomiting). There's also a long list of drugs that may possibly cause lupus, but researchers lack definite proof of the association. It's thought that about 10 per cent of people with lupus have drug-induced symptoms.

There seems to be a genetic tendency to develop lupus. In families of people with lupus, there is an increased incidence of both lupus and rheumatoid arthritis. That genetic tendency, along with exposure to certain viruses, chemicals in the environment or extreme emotional stress, may trigger the immune process that leads to the formation of antibodies against the self.

Q   **Who gets lupus?**

A   Ninety per cent of lupus patients are female. The disease affects one in 700 white females, and one in 250 black females.

Q   **How is it diagnosed?**

A   The skin rash of discoid lupus may be so typical that its appearance, along with a medical history, is enough to make a diagnosis. Someone with discoid lupus needs to have a complete physical examination, including laboratory tests to check for the possibility of SLE.

Diagnosing SLE is more difficult. A doctor who suspects lupus usually orders several blood tests which can detect various abnormal antibodies. The **antinuclear antibody (ANA) test** is a very useful screening test, because it is positive in at least 99 per cent of people with systemic lupus. However, antinuclear antibodies may also be formed in reaction to certain medications, viral infections, liver diseases and various types of arthritis. So a positive result does not necessarily confirm that you have lupus, though a negative ANA test makes this diagnosis quite unlikely.

The blood test most commonly used to confirm the diagnosis of lupus detects antibodies to a person's own genetic material, DNA. This antibody can be found in the blood of about 75 per cent of people with SLE, but it is rarely present in any other condition.

Q How is lupus treated?

A Discoid lupus may be treated with topical steroid creams and sunscreens. With more extensive skin disease, hydroxychloroquine (Plaquenil), the same anti-malaria drug used to treat rheumatoid arthritis, is sometimes used, and seems to work quite well.

SLE has frequently been treated with long-term high-dose steroid drugs. But the great majority of experts now say that most patients on high-dose steroids are paying too dearly for relief. Kidney failure and heart disease, the two conditions most likely to lead to death in people with lupus, have both been linked with the long-term use of steroid drugs. So experts recommend that steroids should not be used unless major organs are immediately threatened with inflammation and destruction during disease flare-ups, and then only at the lowest effective dose. Less powerful drugs, including aspirin, nonsteroidal anti-inflammatory drugs (NSAIDs) and antimalaria drugs, can often control symptoms well enough. Or, in some cases, drugs that suppress the immune system may be used.

Q **What is juvenile rheumatoid arthritis?**
A Juvenile rheumatoid arthritis, or Still's disease, is arbitrarily considered to be any kind of arthritis that begins before age 16. Juvenile rheumatoid arthritis is rare before the age of six months, and two onset peaks are generally observed, between the ages of one and three years and between 8 and 12 years. Girls are twice as likely as boys to develop it. In Britain, the prevalence is one in every 1,500 schoolchildren.

The symptoms of juvenile rheumatoid arthritis vary, and the disease is usually divided into three types: pauciarticular, polyarticular and systemic.

Q **What's the difference?**
A Pauciarticular arthritis means arthritis in only a few joints. This is the most common type of Still's disease, accounting for 40 to 50 per cent of cases. In children aged five or older, mild joint pain and swelling are often the only

symptoms. Children who are five or younger may also be listless and irritable, have a low-grade fever and fail to grow at a normal rate. One potentially serious manifestation of this type of arthritis is an inflammation of the iris of the eye, called anterior uveitis, which occurs in 20 to 30 per cent of children. Children with this disorder need to have their eyes checked at least every three months by an ophthalmologist.

Polyarticular juvenile arthritis accounts for 30 to 40 per cent of all cases of Still's disease. It is characterized by arthritis in more than four joints and can begin either abruptly or slowly. In either case, the child appears listless. He or she may refuse to eat and, subsequently, lose weight. Large joints, such as the knees, wrists, ankles and elbows, are the most frequent sites of initial inflammation. The child may also have a low-grade fever, which may peak twice a day at no more than 40°C (102°F).

Systemic juvenile rheumatoid arthritis, the least common type and the one type more likely to affect boys than girls, accounts for about 20 per cent of cases of juvenile rheumatoid arthritis. Its initial symptoms can vary. Sometimes there is simply joint pain, fever and a fleeting rash. In other cases there may be high fever, a rash, enlarged lymph glands and spleen, and often heart and lung inflammation.

Q **What happens to children who develop juvenile rheumatoid arthritis?**

A The overall prognosis for children with Still's disease is better than previously assumed. At least 75 per cent eventually have long remissions without significant residual damage. Children with rheumatoid-factor positive or systemic-onset juvenile RA are at greatest risk of chronic and destructive joint damage. Growth retardation occurs most frequently in children with chronic systemic arthritis or polyarticular arthritis.

Q   **Is juvenile rheumatoid arthritis treated the same way as adult RA?**

A   Not always. Nonsteroidal anti-inflammatory drugs, especially ibuprofen or aspirin, are the mainstays of treatment. Gold therapy may be started in children who haven't responded to NSAIDs within six months. Studies show that the toxicity in children is similar to that in adults and is of no greater severity or frequency. Hydroxychloroquine (Plaquenil) is sometimes used as an alternative to gold. Steroids drugs are avoided except in the case of life-threatening inflammation. Other drugs, such as methotrexate, have not been adequately studied in children. Many doctors think these drugs are too risky to use, since most children with juvenile RA eventually go into remission with little permanent joint damage.

Q   **What is scleroderma?**

A   Scleroderma is a relatively rare form of arthritis that affects women three to four times more often than men, and its incidence increases steadily with age, most commonly with onset between ages 30 and 60.

   Its name comes from the Greek word *sklero*, meaning hard, and *derma*, meaning skin. Many people with the disease develop areas of thick, rigid skin on their faces, fingers and arms. This disease is also called *progressive systemic sclerosis*, because it sometimes involves progressive hardening of tissue in other areas of the body, including the joints, lungs, heart, kidneys and intestinal tract.

Scleroderma is a **collagen vascular disease**. Collagen is the fibrous structural protein that gives resilience to skin and bones and which supports and connects other tissues in the body. In scleroderma the body makes too much collagen, and the excess is deposited in the skin and other organs, resulting in hardness and tightness of the skin and possible organ dysfunction. The disease can also cause the abnormal growth of cells lining the blood vessels, which can cause vascular problems such as the extreme sensitivity of the fingers to cold, a condition called *Raynaud's phenomenon*. The cause of this abnormal collagen growth is unknown. Like lupus, scleroderma is associated with abnormal antibodies which cause the body to attack its own tissue.

Q **What are the symptoms of scleroderma?**

A In most people, the first symptom is either Raynaud's phenomenon, with finger swelling, puffiness and colour changes in response to cold; or pain and swelling in the joints of the hands. Skin thickening usually follows and may spread to other areas of the body. If joints, tendons and muscles become involved, pain, weakness and nerve compression may result. The gastrointestinal tract is frequently involved, and may cause swallowing problems, stomach pain and bloating. Changes in the lungs occur in about 40 per cent of people, but few are incapacitated by this. Heart and kidney problems can also occur, and can be serious.

Q **How is scleroderma diagnosed?**
A There is no single test for this disease. Your doctor may order blood tests to rule out some other forms of arthritis and to check for certain types of antibodies. He or she may do tests to check the function of your lungs, heart, kidneys and gastrointestinal tract.

Q **How is scleroderma treated?**
A No single drug or combination of drugs has been demonstrated to be effective in controlling scleroderma. The use of steroids is usually restricted to severe inflammation. Immunosuppressive drugs have been tried, but reports of their effectiveness have been inconsistent. Nonsteroidal anti-inflammatory drugs are sometimes given to treat the arthritis symptoms associated with scleroderma. Drugs that dilate blood vessels may be used to improve circulation in tiny blood vessels and to help prevent high blood pressure and kidney damage. Heartburn may be treated with antacids, and problems with digesting and absorbing foods may mean you'll need to drink special nutrient-packed drinks.

Like rheumatoid arthritis, the course of scleroderma varies considerably. Overall, the 10-year survival rate after first diagnosis is approximately 65 per cent. The prognosis for this disease continues to improve, however, with the use of effective blood-pressure drugs which reduce the incidence of kidney failure.

Q **Haven't silicone breast implants been associated with scleroderma and rheumatoid arthritis?**

A Silicone breast implants may be associated with some connective-tissue diseases, but one study reported no increased numbers of women with breast implants in a group of women with scleroderma. Most of the evidence which would connect silicone breast implants with scleroderma consists of anecdotal reports and reports of improvement in symptoms after breast implants are removed. The most common symptoms associated with silicone breast implants seem to be fatigue and muscle and joint pain.

More than 25,000 lawsuits in the US led authorities there to ban silicone breast implants in 1992. The manufacturers have had to pay over $3 billion into a legal settlement fund. None of this is scientific evidence that silicone causes these diseases. The difficulty is to prove a causal relationship. The manufacturers, and many scientists, remain sceptical.

INFORMATION AND
MUTUAL AID GROUPS

The Arthritic Association
Hill House
Little New Street
London W1X 8HB
0171–491 0233

Arthritis Care
18 Stephenson Way
London NW1 2HD
0171–916 1500
Free helpline 0800 289170

Arthritis and Rheumatism Council
25 Bradiston Road
London W9 3HN
0181–964 5590

British Association of Occupational Therapists
6 Marshalsea Road
London SE1 1TV
0171–357 6480

The British Chiropractic Association
Premier House
10 Greycoat Place
London SW1P 1SB
0171–222 8866

Council for Acupuncture
179 Gloucester Place
London NW1 6VX
0171–724 5756

Disabled Living Foundation
380–384 Harrow Road
London W9 2HU
0171–289 6111

GLOSSARY

ACETAMINOPHEN

A pain-relieving and fever-reducing drug used in many over-the-counter remedies

ACUPUNCTURE

An ancient Chinese healing art that involves inserting very thin needles into certain points along the body to relieve pain and promote healing

ACUTE

Beginning quickly; sharp or severe

ANAEMIA

A reduction to below-normal in the number of red blood cells in the blood or in the haemoglobin within the cells. A common symptom of anaemia is fatigue

ANKYLOSING SPONDYLITIS

A type of arthritis which primarily affects the spine and sacroiliac joints. **Tendons** and **ligaments** may become inflamed where they attach to the bone. Advanced forms may result in the formation of bony bridges between vertebrae, causing the spine to become rigid

ANTIBODY

A type of blood protein made by the body in response to a foreign substance (**antigen**). An antibody binds to an antigen so that the immune system can eliminate it from the body

ANTIGEN

Any substance the body regards as foreign or potentially dangerous, and which results in the production of an **antibody**

ANTI-INFLAMMATORY DRUG

A drug, such as aspirin or ibuprofen, which reduces pain, redness, swelling and heat

ANTINUCLEAR ANTIBODY (ANA) TEST

A screening test used for several types of inflammatory conditions, and especially useful in detecting **systemic lupus erythematosus**. It is positive in at least 99 per cent of people with systemic lupus. However, antinuclear antibodies may also be formed in reaction to certain drugs, viral infections, liver diseases, various types of arthritis and even ageing

ARTHRODESIS

Fixing a joint through surgery to relieve pain or give support; fusion

ARTHROSCOPE

A flexible viewing tube about the diameter of a pencil, inserted through a small incision into the **joint capsule**, which provides a view of the inside of a joint and allows for surgery

ARTHROSCOPIC SURGERY

Surgery done on a joint using an **arthroscope**

GLOSSARY

ARTICULAR
>Pertaining to a joint

ATROPHY
>Decrease in the size of a normally developed organ or tissue; wasting

AUTOIMMUNE DISEASE
>A disease due to the action of the immune system against the body tissues, occurring because the immune cells can't differentiate between the body's own material ('self') and that which is foreign ('non-self'). It is possible that certain body proteins are so altered by viral infections, by combination with a drug or chemical, or by other means, that they are no longer recognizable by the body as 'self' and therefore are rejected as foreign

BIOLOGICAL AGENT
>A laboratory-produced substance, similar to the body's own biochemicals and administered in the same manner as drugs, which alters the body's immune response

BONE SPUR
>A bony growth around the joints seen in people with **osteoarthritis**. Joints may appear to be swollen, and pressure on the spur may cause pain

BURSITIS
>**Inflammation** of the bursas, small, fluid-filled sacs which cushion and reduce friction where muscles and **tendons** move over bones or **ligaments**, such as in the shoulders, hips, knees and elbows

CARPAL TUNNEL SYNDROME
>A group of symptoms resulting from compression of the medial nerve in the wrist, with pain and burning or

tingling numbness in the fingers and hand, sometimes extending to the elbow

CARTILAGE

A smooth, resilient tissue which covers the ends of the bones so they don't rub against each other

CHONDROITIN SULPHATE

A product, available in some health-food stores, which contains **glycosaminoglycans**, major structural components of **cartilage** and **connective tissue**. Although this product is popular, there are no scientific reasons to believe that it helps to rebuild cartilage

CHROMOSOME

One of 46 structures in the nucleus of every cell containing genetic material which determines the characteristics of the body

CHRONIC

Persisting for a long time

COLCHICINE

A drug used in the treatment of gout, usually effective in terminating an attack of gout; side-effects may include gastrointestinal symptoms and low blood pressure

COLLAGEN VASCULAR DISEASE

An **autoimmune disease** in which the body's fibrous collagen tissues and the cells lining the inside of blood vessels overgrow, causing organ dysfunction and circulation problems

COMPLETE BLOOD COUNT

A diagnostic test which measures blood components, including white blood cells, red blood cells and **platelets**. Sometimes also called a full blood count

GLOSSARY

COMPUTERIZED AXIAL TOMOGRAPHIC SCAN (A CT OR CAT SCAN)

A sophisticated x-ray imaging technique which produces thin cross-sectional images of body organs

CONNECTIVE TISSUE

A long-fibre type of body tissue which supports and connects internal organs, forms bones and the walls of blood vessels, attaches muscles to bone, and replaces tissues of other types following injury

CORTISONE (CORTICOSTEROID)

A potent and effective steroid drug related to the hormone cortisol, produced by the adrenal glands. Steroid drugs quickly reduce swelling and **inflammation**, but do have possibly serious side-effects

CULTURE

The propagation of micro-organisms or living tissue in a special medium conducive to their growth. Fluid withdrawn from a joint might be cultured to see what micro-organisms, if any, it contains

CYCLOSPORINE

A drug used to prevent rejection in organ transplant patients, used with some success in people with **rheumatoid arthritis** who haven't responded well to other treatments

CYST

An enclosed sac or capsule in the body which contains fluid or a semi-solid material. Although harmless, a cyst can become infected

DEEP HEAT

A treatment which uses tissue-penetrating **ultrasound**

waves to heat up small areas of the body; the only heat treatment which can penetrate beyond the surface layers of the skin to a joint

DEGENERATIVE JOINT DISEASE

Another name for **osteoarthritis**

DISCOID LUPUS

A form of lupus which affects only the skin, causing a rash usually across the face and upper part of the body

DISEASE-MODIFYING

Altering, changing or slowing the course of a disease

DISEASE-REMITTIVE

Altering, changing or slowing the course of a disease

DMSO (DIMETHYL SULPHOXIDE)

A solvent which is sometimes applied to swollen, painful joints. There is no convincing evidence that it is effective

ECHOCARDIOGRAM

A test which uses sound waves to detect fluid around the heart and other heart abnormalities

EICOSAPENTAENOIC ACID

Omega-3 fatty acids found in fish such as mackerel, sardines and salmon and shown to inhibit **inflammation** in the body

ERYTHROCYTE SEDIMENTATION RATE

A test which measures how fast red blood cells cling together, fall, and settle to the bottom of a narrow tube. The more inflammatory proteins found in the blood, the faster these cells clump together and sink in a period of one hour

FASTING

Abstaining from food

FIBROMYALGIA

A disease involving pain in muscles or joints with no clinical signs of **inflammation**

FIBROUS

Composed of or containing fibres. **Ligaments**, for instance, are rubbery bands of strong fibrous tissue

FLARE-UP

A period of time when symptoms worsen

GAMMA-INTERFERON

A medicinal preparation, derived from live cells, which is being tried experimentally in the treatment of RA and other **rheumatic diseases**. A biochemical produced by certain of the body's immune cells, gamma-interferon has a range of effects on the body's immune system

GAMMA-LINOLENIC ACID

A fatty acid, found in high concentrations in blackcurrant oil, evening-primrose oil and borage oil, and thought to have anti-inflammatory actions in the body

GENETIC MARKERS

Specific genes or groups of genes on **chromosomes** which indicate a particular genetic tendency, including a tendency to develop certain types of diseases

GLYCOSAMINOGLYCANS

The major structural components of **cartilage** and **connective tissue**. Available as **chondroitin sulphate**

GOLD SALTS

Gold compounds, given by injection or orally, used in the treatment of **rheumatoid arthritis**

GOUT

A form of arthritis caused by deposits of uric acid

crystals in the joint. Gout usually strikes a single joint, often the big toe and often with sudden, severe pain

HAEMATOCRIT

The volume percentage of red blood cells in whole blood

HAEMOGLOBIN

An iron-protein compound which transports oxygen in the blood

HAEMORRHAGE

The escape of blood from a ruptured vessel. Haemorrhage can be external, internal or into the skin or other tissues

HYDROXYCHLOROQUINE

An antimalaria drug (trade name **Plaquenil**) which is used to treat **rheumatoid arthritis**

IBUPROFEN

A widely-used **nonsteroidal anti-inflammatory** agent

IMMUNOSUPPRESSIVE

Inhibiting the immune system in a way which interferes with the formation of antibodies

IMMUNOTOXIN

A **monoclonal antibody** which contains a toxin. The antibody kills a targeted immune cell and thus represses **inflammation**

INFECTIOUS ARTHRITIS

A type of arthritis caused by an infection somewhere in the body. The infection travels to the joint

INFLAMMATION

The body's protective response to an injury or infection. The classic signs – heat, redness, swelling and pain – are produced as a result of biochemicals secreted by the body's infection-fighting immune cells as they attempt to wall off and destroy any germs, and to break down and remove damaged tissue

JOINT CAPSULE

A tough, fibrous, fluid-filled tissue which completely surrounds a joint. A **synovial membrane** lining the joint capsule secretes fluid which keeps the joint lubricated

JUVENILE RHEUMATOID ARTHRITIS

Any type of arthritis which develops in children. Often known as Still's disease. There are several subtypes

LIGAMENT

A thick, cordlike fibre which attaches to bones to keep them in correct alignment

LIVER BIOPSY

A surgical procedure to remove a small sample of liver tissue for examination. The tissue is procured using a long, hollow-core needle, inserted through the skin into the liver

LUPUS

See **Systemic lupus erythematosus**

LYME DISEASE

A type of arthritis caused by the bacteria *Borrelia burgdorferi* transmitted by a tick which infests a variety of animals, including deer, mice and domestic animals such as dogs

LYMPHOMA

Cancer of the lymph glands, which are part of the immune system

MAGNETIC RESONANCE IMAGING (MRI)

A non-invasive medical procedure that can produce images of soft tissues which would not be seen on an x-ray

MAST CELL

A type of immune cell, often found on the surface linings of organs, that is involved in allergic reactions

METHOTREXATE

A powerful drug, with many potential side-effects, used in the treatment of **rheumatoid arthritis**

MINOCYCLINE

A form of the antibiotic tetracycline currently being tested in a clinical trial as a treatment for **rheumatoid arthritis**

MONOCLONAL ANTIBODY

A laboratory-produced antibody being used experimentally to diminish inflammatory reactions in the body

NEURITIS

Inflammation of the nerves

NIGHTSHADE

A botanical family which includes potatoes, eggplants, tomatoes, peppers (red and green bell peppers, chili peppers and paprika) and which some people believe can cause joint **inflammation**

NITRATES

Food preservatives found in cured meats and some other foods which may cause joint swelling in some people

NONSTEROIDAL ANTI-INFLAMMATORY DRUGS (NSAIDS)

A group of drugs having pain-relieving, fever-reducing and anti-inflammatory effects due to their ability to inhibit the synthesis of **prostaglandins**. Includes aspirin, **ibuprofen** and many prescription drugs

OMEGA-3 FATTY ACID

Also called **eicosapentaenoic acid**, a fatty acid found in fish such as mackerel, sardines and salmon, and shown to inhibit **inflammation** in the body

ORTHOPAEDIC SPECIALIST (OR ORTHOPAEDIC SURGEON)

A doctor who specializes in surgery of the bones, joints and related structures

OSCILLOSCOPE

An instrument which displays a visual representation of electrical variations on a fluorescent screen

OSTEOARTHRITIS

Degenerative arthritis, often caused by joint injuries or old age. The most common type of arthritis

OSTEONECROSIS

Death of bone cells

PENICILLAMINE

A drug, related to penicillin, which is sometimes used to treat **rheumatoid arthritis**

PERICARDITIS

Inflammation of the pericardium, the fibrous tissue surrounding the heart

PLACEBO

An inert substance, often in the form of a lactose tablet

or injection of sterile water, which may be given under the guise of effective treatment. In 'controlled' clinical research studies, a group of people taking a placebo is compared with a group receiving the treatment being studied. The placebo group is called the 'control group'. Studies show that about one-third of people taking a placebo – for any reason – show an improvement in symptoms, at least initially. This phenomenon is called the 'placebo response'

PLAQUENIL

Brand name for an antimalaria drug (**hydroxychloroquine**) which is also used to treat **rheumatoid arthritis**

PLATELET

A very small blood element, a fragment of a larger cell, which aggregates with its fellows, tends to adhere to damaged or uneven surfaces and initiates the clotting of blood

PROSTAGLANDIN

A hormone-like substance produced in the body from fatty acids. Prostaglandins form a varied family and have a variety of effects, including the control of and causation of **inflammation**

PURINE

A protein compound, found in anchovies, organ meats, mushrooms and other foods, which can aggravate gout by elevating body levels of uric acid, which crystallizes in joints

RANGE-OF-MOTION EXERCISE

Exercise designed specifically to keep a joint flexible

REMISSION

Diminution or abatement of the symptoms of a disease

REVISION

An operation to repair or replace an artificial joint which has loosened, broken or become infected

RHEUMATIC DISEASE

A condition which involves **inflammation** and degeneration of **connective tissues** and related structures. Such diseases can affect the joints, muscles, **tendons** and **ligaments**, heart and lungs, skin and eyes, as well as the protective coverings of some internal organs

RHEUMATOID ARTHRITIS

A chronic disease with inflammatory changes occurring throughout the body's **connective tissues**

RHEUMATOID FACTOR

An auto-antibody of the IgM class, found in the blood of many people with **rheumatoid arthritis**, which combines with a commoner type of antibody to form complexes which are implicated in the joint **inflammation**

RHEUMATOID NODULE

A small round or oval bump just under the skin found in some people with **rheumatoid arthritis**

RHEUMATOLOGIST

A doctor who specializes in the treatment of arthritis, especially **rheumatoid arthritis** and other inflammatory diseases

SACROILIAC JOINTS

The joints between the tailbone (sacrum) – five fused vertebrae – and the side bones of the pelvis

SCLERODERMA

A condition which involves thickening of the skin and changes in blood vessels and the immune system

SOLANINE

A chemical substance found in plants such as tomatoes and potatoes. In large amounts, solanine may produce joint **inflammation**

SPLINT

A rigid or flexible appliance to immobilize or protect inflamed joints

STERNUM

The plate of bones forming the breastbone

STEROID DRUG

A class of potent drugs related to the hormone cortisol, produced by the adrenal glands. Steroid drugs quickly reduce swelling and **inflammation**, but have possible serious side-effects

SUBCHONDRAL BONE

Bone found directly under the **cartilage** of a joint

SULPHASALAZINE

A powerful drug used in the treatment of **rheumatoid arthritis**. In a preliminary study by Dutch researchers, sulphasalazine (Salazopyrin) was found to slow joint destruction in people with early RA

SYMMETRICAL

Equal in size or shape (of the parts on either side of the body); very similar in placement about an axis

SYNOVECTOMY

The cutting-out of a **synovial membrane** of a joint

SYNOVIAL FLUID

Fluid secreted by the synovium, the cells lining a **joint capsule**, which lubricates the joint and helps nourish the **cartilage**

SYNOVIAL MEMBRANE

The synovium. The cells lining the inside of the **joint capsule**, which secrete lubricating fluid. In **rheumatoid arthritis**, the synovial membrane overgrows the joint capsule, invades the **cartilage**, and begins to secrete biochemicals which can destroy a joint

SYNOVIUM

See **Synovial membrane**

SYSTEMIC LUPUS ERYTHEMATOSUS (SLE)

A chronic, body-wide inflammatory condition which affects the joints, skin, blood, lungs, cardiovascular and nervous systems and kidneys

TENDON

A strong band of tissue which connects muscle to bone

TENDINITIS

Inflammation of a **tendon**

TRANSDUCER

A device which translates one physical quantity, such as pressure or temperature, to an electrical signal

TRIPTERGIUM WILFORDII (THUNDERVINE ROOT)

A Chinese herbal remedy for **rheumatoid arthritis** currently undergoing clinical trials in China

ULTRASOUND

A technique in which deep structures of the body are visualized by recording the reflections (echoes) of ultrasonic waves directed into the tissues

URIC ACID CRYSTALS
   Tiny, needle-shaped particles which form in a joint when concentrations of uric acid become high, as in gout

VASCULITIS
   Inflammation of blood vessels

VEGAN DIET
   A vegetarian diet which excludes dairy products and eggs

USEFUL REFERENCES

'Arthritis in children', *British Medical Journal*, 18 March 1995: 728

'Arthritis joint disease review', *Doctor*, 5 April 1990: 39

'Bone loss in rheumatoid arthritis', *Lancet*, 2 July 1994: 3, 23

'Borrelia in joints', *New England Journal of Medicine*, January 27 1994: 229

'Cartilage culture for joint surgery', *New Scientist*, 29 October 1994: 25

'Collagen collagenase and arthritis', *New Scientist*, 8 June 1991: 39

'Folklore remedies for arthritis', *Pulse*, 14 April 1990: 91

'Immunology and joint disease arthritis', *New Scientist*, 4 May 1991: 40

'Joint cracking can cause damage', *British Medical Journal*, 23/30 December 1989: 1566

'Knee-joint replacement', *Lancet*, 22 November 1986: 1196

'MRI of joint disease', *British Journal of Hospital Medicine*, 2 February 1994: 97

'Musician joint hypermobility', *New England Journal of Medicine*, October 7 1993: 1079

'Osteoarthritis', *British Medical Journal*, 18 February 1995: 457

'Rest or exercise in arthritis', *British Journal of Hospital Medicine*, 21 October 1992: 445

'Rheumatoid arthritis and the drug Colloral', *New Scientist*, 14 May 1994: 19

'Rheumatoid arthritis, features and diagnosis', *British Medical Journal*, 4 March 1995: 587

'Rheumatoid arthritis, infectious disease?', *British Medical Journal*, 17 July 1991: 200

'Rheumatoid arthritis management', *British Medical Journal*, 14 August 1993: 425

'Rheumatoid arthritis management review', *British Journal of Hospital Medicine*, 1–28 July 1992: 106

'Rheumatoid arthritis path management', *Lancet*, 30 January 1993: 283, 286

'Rheumatoid arthritis treatment with cyclosporine and methotrexate', *New England Journal of Medicine*, July 20 1995: 137, 183

'Spinal joint problems', *British Medical Journal*, 20 May 1995: 1321

'Steroids and joint destruction in rheumatoid arthritis', *New England Journal of Medicine*, July 20 1995: 142, 183

'Taping patella knee osteoarthritis', *British Medical Journal*, 19 March 1994: 753

'Temporomandibular joint replacement', *British Journal of Hospital Medicine*, 3 May 1995: 455

'Treating rheumatoid arthritis', *British Medical Journal*, 11 March 1995: 652

'Vegetarian diet fasting rheumatoid arthritis', *Lancet*, 12 October 1991: 899

INDEX

ARTHRITIS

Of further interest…

ARTHRITIS

ALLERGY, NUTRITION AND THE ENVIRONMENT

Dr John Mansfield

All major forms of arthritis are related to allergy, the environment and nutrition. Recent research has led to a greater understanding of the role nutrition has in the treatment of arthritis — both in reducing chemical sensitivity and food allergy. Dr Mansfield argues against suppressing symptoms with drugs, outlining exactly what action sufferers of arthritis can take to tackle the cause of illness. He explains:

- the importance of essential fatty acids, trace minerals, B vitamins and other nutrients
- environmental and food allergens and their effect
- the damaging effect of drugs on the body's immune system
- the link with candida albicans and advice to sufferers
- finding a diagnosis — including elimination diets and skin testing

DIETS TO HELP: ARTHRITIS

Helen Macfarlane

Many thousands of people have found that simple changes to their diet can help alleviate the pain and discomfort which are symptomatic of arthritis.

- low fat
- low protein
- low carbohydrate

This book offers simple dietary guidelines to help correct the nutritional balance of the body. It explains:

- the role of fruit and vegetables
- why you should reduce protein foods
- the trouble with refined carbohydrates
- how to reduce mucus-forming foods

It also features a selection of basic recipes, advice on vitamins and minerals and explains the role of the Hay System of eating.

ARTHRITIS	0 7225 1903 6	£6.99	☐
DIETS TO HELP: ARTHRITIS	0 7225 2871 X	£2.99	☐

All these books are available from your local bookseller or can be ordered direct from the publishers.

To order direct just tick the titles you want and fill in the form below:

Name: _____

Address: _____

_____

_____ Postcode: _____

Send to Thorsons Mail Order, Dept 3, HarperCollins*Publishers*, Westerhill Road, Bishopbriggs, Glasgow G64 2QT.
Please enclose a cheque or postal order or your authority to debit your Visa/Access account –

Credit card no: _____

Expiry date: _____

Signature: _____

– up to the value of the cover price plus:
UK & BFPO: Add £1.00 for the first book and 25p for each additional book ordered.
Overseas orders including Eire: Please add £2.95 service charge. Books will be sent by surface mail but quotes for airmail dispatches will be given on request.

24-HOUR TELEPHONE ORDERING SERVICE FOR ACCESS/VISA CARDHOLDERS — TEL: 0141 772 2281.